How to do Low Carb, UK style!

UK style!

Eat your way to an optimal body

How to do Low Carb, UK style!

UK style!

Eat your way to an optimal body

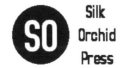

Silk
Orchid
Press

.

How to do Low Carb, UK Style!

No part of this book may be produced by any means, nor transmitted, nor translated into a machine language, without the written permission of the publisher.

The right of Nikola Howard to be identified as the author of this work has been asserted in accordance with sections 77 and 78 of the Copyright, Designs & Patent Act 1988

CONDITIONS OF SALE: This book is sold subject to the condition that it shall not, by way of trade or otherwise, be lent, resold, hired out, or otherwise circulated without the publisher's prior consent in any form of binding or cover other than that in which it is published and without a similar condition, including this condition, being imposed on the subsequent purchaser.

First Published by Silk Orchid Press in The United Kingdom of Great Britain and Northern Ireland in 2018.

Paperback Edition ISBN 978-1-9164409-0-6

This first edition published in August 2018 by Nikola Howard

"As long as you consider a 'short term diet as a solution', you are doomed to an 'on-again, off-again' battle with your weight"

-   Dr Robert C. Atkins

Introduction

'Food is not just calories, it is information. It talks to your DNA and tells it what to do. The most powerful tool to change your health, environment and entire world is your fork."

- Dr Mark Hyman

Hello, welcome and thank you - thank you for picking up this book, asking me to help you and acknowledging to yourself that you might need a little help with dropping some fat and gaining your optimal body.

Have you tried every diet going and then some? Have you found that you diet for a while, only to crash out after a few months, and then put on more weight than you took off? Do you feel self-hate because you "cannot stick to a diet" or because you cannot seem to achieve the same look as other women in fashion and women's magazines?

The dietary advice offered in the mainstream since the 1980's is a diet based around keeping overall calories low and eating mostly carbohydrates - a diet that works against the way our bodies evolved - and causes constant hunger, messes with our brain chemistry to cause sugar cravings and reduces the speed of our metabolism.

This advice fails us because it teaches us to belittle and ignore natural biological signals of hunger and to use willpower to resist eating enough food. This setup causes feelings of failure as willpower is a finite resource that we cannot use constantly. It also causes feeling of deprivation and resentment.

Whilst government and the medical profession say that the standard western diet is the best way to eat, the media and society continually tells us that if we don't comply with a diet that causes constant hunger that we are weak-willed and implies that it's all our fault and that we deserve to be fat and unhealthy.

Even when we do comply (and feel miserable whilst doing so), when we remain fat whilst eating less and less (especially if we have the body type that likes to store fat), we judge ourselves and presume that (usually skinny) people assume that we must be "cheating" or "not trying hard enough".

This constant self-judgment sets up a mentality of "being good" and "being bad" in our mind, and when we do eat more food than we are told we are allowed, or we eat something that is seen as "bad for us" we feel guilty as hell and hate ourselves for doing so, when all we are doing is simply responding to what our body is crying out for, food. This puts us at war with ourselves and produces nothing but a society filled with anguish and self-hatred.

I want to set you free from this cycle. I'm on a one-woman mission to remove the linguistically horrific words "weight loss" from common usage. My crazy idea is to improve the world by helping others free their minds from self-hate and their bodies from slavery to carbohydrate addiction.

In this book, I am going to present to you not only a new way of eating but also a paradigm shift to a new way of thinking.

I want to reunite your body and your mind so that we create a "happy you" - one that feels that you're deserving of goodness, success and love in life. I am going to challenge you and all your current knowledge about eating, dieting and living life to the full. I'll acknowledge, this can be a scary thought, so I'm going to thank you again for your bravery in picking up this book and not putting it down again having read the last paragraph!

Just like you, I tried all the calories restricted diets going and suffered hunger, tiredness, mood swings and self-hate because of them. I found low carbohydrate eating in 1999 and discovered that a diet based around fat and protein removes hunger and also effortlessly removes body fat.

I was looking for "yet another diet", instead I found a way of eating that could become a happy and successful way of life.

Because I'm a logic-based problem solver, I also delved deeply into the "why" of how our bodies work and therefore why our current paradigm really isn't working for us. I also discovered how we've been let down by some close-minded, biased and decidedly non-scientific scientists influencing government.

The first part of the book is all about the nine shifts that we make in order to end up eating Low Carb, UK style. If you do no more than read and implement this first part of the book, you will be good to go. If you stop here, good luck to you and I wish you well.

However, I do hope that you stick around for part two, (or even read it first!) because if changing food on its own worked, then **any** diet would result in long term success for everyone. Yet we know that the majority of "dieters" go back to their previous weight (and more) within 2 years of achieving their goal weight.

So, to have long terms success, we also need to make crucial shifts in our thinking to break negative and pejorative messaging around food and the cycle of society-imposed self-hate around our bodies, and so affect permanent change to ourselves.

In part two, I'm going hand you the ten keys that will allow you to gently disengage your self-worth as being defined as a number on a weighing scale and embed a new way of thinking - I'm going to introduce you to the concept of optimal, and how that applies to food, your body, your mind and your life.

An optimal body is what you define as optimal for **you** - it could be the size of your waist, what dress size you want to be, how much weight you can bench or how big your biceps are. It could simply be a feeling of rightness in your own skin. The key with optimal is that you get to choose. We're also going to take a tour through what language we use to describe the journey we take to get to our optimal body.

As we work through this book together, we're going to get rid of the limiting language and assumptions that we don't even know holds us back - the casual (or not so casual) words we use that send conflicting signals to our subconscious. There is also a whole bunch of things that our parents, friends and society have told us we are - all of which form heavy chains around our thoughts, because we simply assumed what they said to us was true.

We're going to get subversive and show ourselves lots of love. After all, self-hate is the default position we are taught to have about ourselves and changing this is a major key to our long-term happiness.

Reclaiming our optimal body and optimal self is all about honouring ourselves with optimal choices. Without a change to our habits, we stand no chance at all in keeping the optimal body toward which we are working. To retain and keep an optimal body, we need a revolution with our relationship with food - we need to change not only the way we eat but the way we think.

As T. Harv Eker said *'Where focus goes, energy flows and results show"* - when our "self-talk" is a constant refrain of "oh my gosh I'm so fat / ugly / poor / stupid" then that's exactly what we are, because that is where our focus is.

Our self-talk reflecting negative assumptions about our current state keeps our reality trapped in that state. Simply put, this type of self-talk is self-hate. Given to us by other people opinions, the habit of self-hate forms and reinforces itself over time.

We would never accept anyone else talking to us in this manner, yet we do it to ourselves all the time!

Habits form as we do something over and over and over. The subconscious learns the pattern over time and once ingrained, it can effortlessly repeat the pattern without us having to consciously think about it.

For instance, brushing our teeth is a habit, and so using a knife and fork, walking, talking, typing, writing and driving a car. It's also the late-night fridge grazing, the mindless eating whilst sitting in front of the telly and the being focused on our problems rather than working towards the solution.

So, we will look at our habits, and see how our negative ones are holding us in place and how we can work to change them. *'I have decided to stick with love. Hate is too great a burden to bear"* is a good statement to remember, said by Martin Luther King.

I'll give you plenty of tools to support the change, a printables supplement full of recipe as well as a free subliminal audio track that will help you to put your mind into a better place. Details on how to obtain the latter two are at the back of the book.

In part three, I'll take you for a spin through the science behind this way of life.

Although there are small sprinklings of science through both parts one and two (as without this, you may not understand why you are doing something, and so may find it harder to do it), I've left the lion's share of the science until later, and you don't have to read this part to have success.

However, many people will question, and some will outright attack you for starting to eat in a low carb way, and so having the reasons to hand as to why this way of eating is healthier for the body than the way we are told to eat is a good thing.

Finally, we will go over the UK specific stuff, such as our labelling laws, that so often cause confusion when reading websites from the US, or books that are imported from the US without making the relevant changes to the UK market - the main reason I created http://lowcarbinthe.uk back in 2000!

I'm dedicated to helping you reclaim your optimal body, build an optimal mind and create an optimal you, so that you can enjoy the successes that I and countless others have seen with a low carb way of eating, and I want you to be able to be confident in your choices and able to share the paradigm shift we are creating for the world with others.

What did I learn whilst writing this book?

I learned that, depressingly, the first "reducing diet" was crafted by Hippocrates between 460 and 370 BC, and that throughout modern history, fat is the enemy that must be removed ruthlessly, both from our bodies and our diet.

I also learned that we decided that a person's weight rather than any of their other attributes is the measure of their validity very early in our history, with women taking the brunt of this judgement, but men getting their fair share of the judgement also.

In the last 2000 years, vomiting and drinking vinegar, eating soap, fibre and other digestive interrupters, as well as taking purgatives and various amphetamines or other metabolism raising drugs have been deployed in "the fight against fat".

Another tool used has had us eating "bland foods that did not invite or excite the body to want excess" along with a not so healthy dose of the Abrahamic religious sense that the body must be controlled and denied of food and pleasure so that it remained slender, pure and fit to serve God.

Add in some outright quackery, useless and in some instances dangerous pills, pummelling and corsetry and it feels like my mission is an uphill battle of much bigger proportion than I first thought.

I also learned that all scientists are human; they "cherry pick" data that fits the hypothesis they are trying to prove and that they skew their interpretations to fit the ascendant theories of their time. It is quite rare to find the study that doesn't show any of this very human bias.

I've had to revise a few of my own view points as well because of this, as I try to be as unbiased as I can - but naturally, I'm human as well, and so I have my own bias towards eating in a low carb, moderate protein, high fat way, as it works for me and the many other people I help to achieve their optimal body.

I'll put my hand up now and freely say that this way of eating might well not be for you. After all, we all evolved from different ancestral stock, and this way of eating may well simply not play to the cards that your genetics have dealt you.

Some people run extremely well on a high carb diet, and in fact, in my research I've found quite the mass of studies from the early 20th century that show the fascinatingly similar effects of both an "extreme low fat (sub 10% of diet), low protein and high carb diet" can do almost exactly the same for the body in terms of reduction of body fat, inflammation markers and hormone profile as a "low carb, moderate protein, high fat diet" does.

However, the study subjects in these extremely high carb diets generally had trouble sticking with the protocols due to hunger and lack of variety (rice, rice and more rice was usually the order of the day with these protocols).

So, it's really comes down to what you and your body find more comfortable. All bodies are different, and I advise everyone to treat life as an experiment. Play and learn what "your foods" are and in what amounts your body loves them the best.

If you are reading this book, it's almost certainly because the current "standard diet" advice hasn't worked for you, you are carrying excess body fat and/or quite possibly a host of other disease, such as diabetes, high blood pressure and heart issues.

I firmly believe that if you have the type of body that "fattens easily"[1] – a factor determined by your epigenetic imprint, for instance, whether your great-great-great ancestors survived famine, where the ability to store body fat efficiently would mean a longer life, that a low carbohydrate way of eating is the only diet that is healthy for your body.

The standard advice causes way more issues than it will ever solve, and even in bodies that stay slender with an excess of carbohydrate, their chances of having health issues later in life that we now medicate away, such as

---

[1] Richard MacKarness, Eat Fat and Grow Slim,1958: http://www.ourcivilisation.com/fat/chap1.htm

heartburn, tiredness, headaches as well as diabetes are multiplied by current dietary advice.

One thing on which a great deal of the studies and nutrition books agree is that since "Western society" started to strip foods away from the way that nature built them. Even if the scientists that authored the studies don't like the result they obtained because they don't fit current hypotheses and so try to trivialise or dismiss their findings...

With the advent of food processing, removing fibre and adding processed sugar into our diets from the 1920's, as well as lowering fat and adding more fructose into our diets in the 80's, any society that adopts these principles grows sicker and more and more obese even as they have reduced calorific and particularly fat intake.

So, whilst from the perspective of a low carb life that all forms of sugar are not good for our bodies at all, we'll put a particular spotlight on how our bodies handle fructose later on, as it's uniquely fattening in its own way.

To quote Dr Robert H. Lustig[2], a paediatrician working with obesity in children, and who is at the forefront of the "return to whole food" movement: *'What do the Atkins' diet (which is all fat, no carb) and the Japanese diet (which is all carbs, no fat) have in common? They both eliminate the sugar Fructose"*

---

[2] Sugar: The bitter truth - https://youtu.be/dBnniua6-oM

My story

So, who am I to be writing this book then?

I am a tall person, always have been. I was a slender baby, 58cm (1ft 11in) long at birth, always the tallest person in my class, and developed into a woman standing 179cm (5ft 11) with size 44 (10) feet.

I started gaining body fat when I hit puberty in 1982. Knowing what I know now, I put this down to my body being of the "fatten easily" type, and my diet including many biscuits and sweets, much ice-cream and my favourite breakfast, dinner and tea - peanut butter on toast.

As I got chubbier, I also had a decreasing desire to do exercise. I was bullied and laughed at during secondary school because of my size and found comfort in carbohydrate based food, adding to the problem.

By 1999, the 121Kg (19st 2lbs) I was carrying around made me a size 26. I didn't really mind, I loved myself as I was. However, around my birthday that year, my health started to make me mind what size my body had got into.

I have some crepitus in my right knee and. carrying around all the excess weight was starting to give me large amounts of pain in the joint. I was also having trouble walking up the stairs at work due to general unfitness and discovered that I had 132cm (52in) hips!

As well as the pain, I was also starting to grow out of the clothes I owned, and my wages at the time didn't permit buying a whole new wardrobe. So, some form of diet was in order.

In the past, I used the typical low-fat diets, with their typical short term "success". My first diet was between 16 and 18, and I dropped from 96Kg (15st 2lbs) to 74Kg (11st 10lbs) with Weight Watchers™ "Exchanges" system; calorie restricted, low-carb, low-fat, moderate protein.

I found all of that weight and added another 25Kg (4st) over the next eleven years, all because I didn't know anything about success mindset at that point in life. During that time, I'd use the Weight Watchers™ "Exchanges" plan intermittently, repeating a yo-yo dieting pattern over and over.

But as a very hypoglycaemic person, the periods of being hungry and ratty whilst "on a diet" were very wearing. When I could, I reached for the raisins as a fast sugar fix, which I saw as my saviour food. Little did I know what the fructose was doing to my body.

As I lost interest in "being on a diet", with its endless restriction on life, the constant draining "No" refrain saw me return to eating whatever I wanted, "big" meals (in terms of calories); Curry, Italian, Greek, Chinese, sweets, ice-cream, biscuits, peanut butter on toast and all the other foods that society deems as bad, naughty or sinful.

What turned my life around from being in "the diet trap" in 1999 was a fella I was working with at that time, Tim. He had recently discovered and used the then new to the UK "Dr Atkins' New Diet Revolution" to drop a substantial amount of weight, and after he described the principles to me, he lent me his copy of the book.

Reading that book changed my life. By removing processed carbohydrate from my life, I discovered freedom from the hunger monster. As a confirmed carnivore anyway, the focus on animal fat and protein meant that I ate the foods I love. There was no sense of deprivation, simply a sense of choice. Life was just better without the sugar and starch.

However, I never reached "goal weight" that first time around. I hit a size 18 and 89Kg (14st 1lb) in 2001, then started a 2-year pattern of being stalled out for about 6 months, then gaining 3Kgs (7lbs), then stalling out again, then gaining another 3Kg (7lbs).

I didn't even think about not being low carb during this time, as I was still getting the other health benefits such as good blood pressure, excellent skin, hair, nails, great muscle tone, regular periods, moderated hunger with no hypoglycaemic symptoms and clear thinking with no tiredness or brain fog.

There was a great deal of turbulence in life however, I was doing overnight shift-work, which meant food was limited to what I could pick up in the local small supermarket, leading to some very non-optimal choices indeed. I was also in an abusive relationship from which I managed to get myself away and then shortly after that I moved to a new house & changed job.

All these things added up to massive stress on the body and to my not counting carbs as carefully as the Atkins' plan demands. So, in mid-2003, I'd got back to a size 22 and up to 106Kg (16st 10lbs) again.

I never thought about giving up though, there was too much good stuff going on with everything else health-wise to simply change away from low-carb; even if I wasn't "getting thin" I was convinced that would come eventually once my life and metabolism sorted itself out.

At that time though, my metabolism was going to take an even bigger hit! Before changing to a low carb way of eating, I'd always had very heavy, lengthy and erratic periods, controlled by being on 'The Pill', and my fat distribution is "apple-shaped" – I have slender arms and legs, no bum or hips to speak of and fat on my body accumulates predominantly around my waist, mid back and stomach.

As I hit my late twenties, what I was reading around Insulin and oestrogen and how that may well be interfering with my "weight loss" made me decide to not use 'The Pill' any more.

However, my periods shortly became longer and longer again, with the bleed lasting around 4-6 weeks at a time. When I had an 8-week period, my GP sent me off to see a specialist. On investigation, my ovaries showed the typical cysts of someone with Polycystic Ovary

Syndrome (PCOS), however, I was diagnosed with endometriosis by the consultant, based on the facts that my hormone profile was picture perfect and there were small spots of endometrial tissue on my sigmoid colon.

He prescribed a 3-month course of Zoladex implant pellets that cause a "mini-menopause" - stopping my ovaries producing oestrogen stone dead and replacing this with Livial oestrogen pills for the last 2 months to prevent bone loss.

The impact to my body and brain of bringing my oestrogen production to a screeching halt was both major and cataclysmic. Almost overnight from the first pellet implant, I started to gain fat and lose my mind, and when the Livial was added, the process accelerated, not helped by the fact that I started self-medicating with sugar, as my brain was screaming for something to just stop the crazy.

Three months later; a whole bunch of tears cried, random eating and "crazy-mad-angst" had happened. I landed up 117Kg (18st 7lbs). Over the course of 2004, even as I tried to get my eating back under control, I gained another 6Kg, (1st), all on my tummy. My Oestrogen/Insulin balance was so out of whack that I don't think I could have avoided gaining that visceral fat.

Back in size 26 clothes, but not quite back inside my mind I was totally held in the thrall of carbs again. My mind came back to some level of normal about a month after stopping the medication, but I'd say that it took most of

2005 and 2006 for my body to settle back down hormonally.

Physically, in the first year after Zoladex/Livial I had no periods at all, then I started a year's worth of pretty much constant menstruation.

There was also a great deal of brain-fog, and tiredness permeated everything I was feeling and doing. I was sleeping 14 hours a day over the weekends and was still dog tired come work on Monday morning.

I'm sure you can guess, I wasn't loving my body, and it wasn't loving me. Despite all my rational brain knew about what food made me feel healthy and happy, I just wasn't in a place where I could stop loving myself with carb laden comfort food.

I didn't have it in me to let go of the spuds and sugar again, they made me feel better, dragged me through the day; that same-ol' same ol' addiction pattern. Now I see that just because you can see the pattern, it doesn't make you less of a person if you cannot step away from it at that time. Back then, I gave myself quite a bit of negative judgement over how weak willed I was.

I was also physically very drained simply from losing so much iron all the time. Time turned, I was able to make minor adjustments to my food, dropping the obvious sweet stuff from life and the brain fog finally started to lift.

I then remembered that my consultant had suggested (but not documented) when I saw him that a Mirena intrauterine system (IUS) be fitted once I'd completed my Zoladex if my periods did not regulate. So, I dragged myself off to the Family Planning Clinic around the corner from work, and after tests and investigations on my womb by the very good NHS nurses there, got my first Mirena fitted in Jan 2007.

From there, things definitely levelled out. I stopped bleeding, started eating better (managed to cut the junk but still not anywhere near to low carb) and the casual affair I started early 2006 sorted itself into a more serious & stable relationship.

One of the things that my then partner got me doing was cycling, and my body loved it! It reshaped, and my muscle tone improved massively. I kept thinking "I really must go low carb and help this muscle building process along!" but I still wasn't ready.

I'd moved to a new house again at the beginning of 2007, and I hated the kitchen. I wasn't ready to spend time in a place I didn't like, to do the cooking that living a low carb live requires. My addict brain hadn't reached its "rock-bottom" yet, it was still finding excuses.

2008 was the year of starting house renovations and some quite horrific back pain. I'm an advocate of the osteopath, having attended on and off since late 2005 for knee pain, usually a few sessions of wonderful clunking and clicking and I'd be sorted and away.

However, December 2007 I managed to give myself a serious L3-L4 Capsular strain, and whilst taking X-rays to ensure I didn't have bone degeneration, we discovered that I have a slight congenital scoliosis and one leg 2cm shorter than the other.

Sorting out the capsular strain and accompanying facet irritation took most of 2008, and of course, during that time, there was no cycling, total house turmoil and no proper thinking about what I was eating either.

2009? Nothing notable changed. The house remained in pieces, and work got manic, with lots of late nights and weekend overtime. Couple that with a hectic social life to distract from the home chaos – being tired from both too much work and too many carbs, I had all the same hypoglycaemic, dry-eyed, dull-skinned problems of the past. I knew the fix, just didn't have the energy to have the motivation to eat properly.

However, from about November 2009, I started cycling again, and finally knew I was ready to be low carb - I just had to find the time to get the carbs out of my system without distraction.

I took the opportunity when my then partner headed off to Holland for a 3-day stag-weekend in March 2010. No one in the house to cook for but me? Nowhere for me to be but at home? Stock up on veggies, steak and cream!!!

I didn't weigh myself when I started again. I didn't really want to know just how bad it had got. I just knew that I was edging out of the size 26's and into the 28's again. I had a 153cm (60in) tummy, and I know that about middle 2009 when the osteopath weighed me I was 124Kg (19st 8lb), so I can only guess it was about the same or a good few kilos north of that.

The second time around, I didn't want to get obsessed with all the numbers. That way madness lies, especially given my hormonal history. Given what I now know about mindset, I believe I made the right choice, as I feel like strict adherence to "the numbers and the counting" is simply re-papering the walls of a diet prison cell. It's the same place as with a low-fat diet, with all the "good and bad, guilt, naughtiness and sin", it just looks different food wise.

I formulated a new approach to how I was going to do low carb, and my results flourished. I chose to eat in a way that I now call "optimally" – avoid the processed carbs & the junk sugars, make sensible choices over the natural suboptimal carbs that have massive antioxidant power, and eat lots of green veg, animal protein & fat to satisfy hunger.

I no longer measure my food, but for writing this book, I analysed my food for a month. I found that I eat between 30-50g of carbohydrate per day. There was also one day where I made quite a few suboptimal and non-optimal choices and I touched 100g. As these types of day are rare, the fat-adapted body can easily deal with the extra glycaemic load.

Living a low carb life is all about making food choices and acknowledge that if a non-optimal higher carb choice is made every now and then, that these can be made and enjoyed without guilt. It is simply a natural part of life. As we make these better, more natural choices we feel better and can relax enough to just let our body take care of the rest.

I formalised my method in 2013, when I discovered mindfulness, and realised that to make a permanent change, I had to change my language as well as the food. I created the three tenets[3] that I'll talk about in the next part of the book and came up with a system of grading my food that totally removes guilt from eating.

The system also gives back the power of choice to the eater. There is no "wagon" to fall off of, it's not "a battle with our weight", it's all simply life and choices made along the way. I started to use this system with my coaching clients in 2015 with much success.

So, I share my approach to low carb with you - we are going to aim to shift permanently into to eating under 100g of carbohydrate a day, and initially aiming at around 50g of carbohydrate a day to promote fat burning. The carbohydrate you choose will mostly come from natural sources that have fibre included.

A low carb life defined as one where we eat no more than 100g of mostly vegetable and lower glycaemic foods per day. You may well find that simply cutting back to 100g is what your body needs. Or, you may be a person that

---

[3] Tenets: the defining principles of your personal journey into this rewarding lifestyle.

need to do a great deal of metabolic healing, and greater carbohydrate restriction is needed to get your body into optimal shape. Around 50g a day is where most people reach their effective fat burning zone, but every body (intentional spacing there) is different.

Either way, being under 100g of carbohydrate a day gives your pancreas a holiday from the amount of Insulin it's pumping out right now and staying at around 50g initially doesn't set you up for later issues with Insulin sensitivity that I believe is caused by starting and staying at 20g of carbohydrate and under over a long time period because a quick result is desired.

My anecdotal research from both myself and from observing many thousands of people eating a low carb diet over the last 18 years has shown that starting your shift to a low carb life with a 20g a day restriction on carbohydrate, as advocated by many authors writing in this area that are interested in giving an initial speedy result, causes many issues later on; long stalls at the same weight and size, and increases in body fat if you eat even slightly over 20g a day.

It's one reason why I'm personally dead set against "being strict Keto" unless there is a medical reason to do so - I'm very much with the late Dr Barry Groves, Mark Sisson and also Dr John Briffa in a more moderate approach.

From what I've seen, I believe that the lower you go to start, the lower you have to stay to keep your body burning its fats away and also the more scale and size stalling you will experience.

I also firmly believe that if you have no medical reason to follow a "medically ketogenic diet" then following one all the time is not at all optimal. It's like taking antibiotics when you aren't sick – it's totally unnecessary and very counterproductive for overall health!

After all, the body is a clever thing, and adapts to whatever we throw at it. I believe that there is more benefit to staying "on the bubble" of mostly ketosis (fat for energy) with a little glucosis (glucose for energy) as it trains the body into becoming metabolically flexible. Which is the way our bodies evolved to work.

This is your way of eating and your way of life, use the information I'm giving you in this book to own it and make it your own.

Part one

How to feed the body optimally so it can live, thrive and survive!

My philosophy is: give the body the right tools and it will look after itself. That way, doctors would only be needed for emergencies and accidents and we could all save a heck of a lot of money and resources that are largely wasted today, and which allow us to be preyed on by the large and avaricious 'health industry'

-       Dr Barry Groves

Why a low carb lifestyle is an easy way of life

One of the reasons that the standard low calorie, low fat diets fail is that they are based around the foods that cause us maximum hunger. A diet based around eating refined carbohydrates (mostly sugar and wheat) that are nutrient sparse means that the digestive mechanisms called on to process them mess with the body's "appestat"[4] - our built-in ability to regulate both our food intake and our hunger.

It also sets up craving pathways in our brain, because the levels of Insulin that the pancreas needs to pump out to cope with all the glucose running around block the brain's ability to sense the glucose made from all starches and most sugars - so, the brain drives you to consume more of these foods because it thinks it is starving!

Before refined carbohydrates our ancestors never had cravings, and it's this "appestat" regulation mechanism that stops wild mammals from becoming obese. By vastly reducing these refined carbohydrates, whilst increasing the nutrient dense foods, fibre, natural fats, protein and vegetables, we begin to run on fat for energy in the main rather than glucose, and the appestat can function appropriately again. This results in diminished cravings and the normal levels of hunger for our species return.

―――――――――――――――――――――

[4]https://realmealrevolution.com/real-thinking/is-your-brain-making-you-fat/

Note that when eating nutrient dense foods, and trusting your body, it will regulate food intake via hunger signals itself – once we learn to recognise these signals, it will mean that most people do not need to restrict their portion sizes at all.

For some people, and especially if you have yo-yo dieted and also have built an "interesting" relationship with food, some overall portion restrictions may be required, but for now, take my word on this. I'll show you more than enough reasons to relax and eat "ad libitum" of protein, fat and most low starch vegetables in the science section later on.

My opinion as to why eating this way is so liberating: You never need to regulate or punish yourself with feeling hungry ever again.

You also don't need to ever feel that you should finish the food in front of you out of obligation or a sense of guilt. If there is still food on your plate when your body tells you that is it satisfied, simply stop eating and stick it in the fridge to eat later.

Also you learn to be aware of "eyes bigger than belly" syndrome – This over loading of the plate habit is mostly built out of being deprived of food by dieting! We shall be working on removing that scarcity mindset later as well.

I've already talked about the concept of optimal, and it applies as much to food as to the rest of your life.

To live an optimal low carb life, follow these three simple tenets:

1) If you are hungry, eat.
2) If you are not hungry, don't eat / stop eating.
3) Make every mouthful as optimal as possible, given the circumstances in which you find yourself.

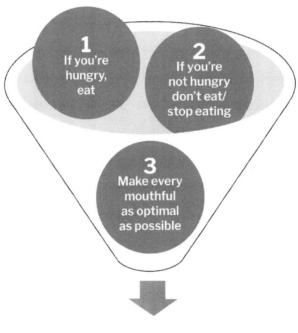

A healthier you

The OSN Scale: What does food in an optimal low carb life look like?

Our food falls into three categories:

Optimal (eat freely - "ad libitum" - and with gusto!):

Plentiful amounts of
- Brassica family vegetables,
  - This is all the "cabbage" family, "green leafy veg" as well as red and white cabbage, broccoli, mustard greens, all the Chinese leaves such as bok choi, choi sum and tatsoi, cauliflower, Brussel sprouts, flower sprouts/kalettes, turnips and turnip greens, swede and swede greens, kohlrabi etc.
  - Fermented vegetables, such as sauerkraut and kimchee, are awesome for your gut heath.
- Meat,
- Fish, especially oily fish,
- Shellfish
- Fowl,
- Game,
- Eggs,
- Hard Cheeses,
- Animal fats such as cream, butter, ghee, lard and dripping,

- ❖ Plant based fats such as coconut oil, olive oil, avocado oil and all nut oils,
- ❖ Avocados
- ❖ All Herbs and "above ground" spices.
- ❖ Beef, Whey, Egg and Pea protein powders
  - ○ The latter three being useful for vegetarians and vegans respectively

Optimal veggies to be eaten with a shade of moderation
- ❖ Vine grown vegetables such as peppers, cucumbers, aubergine, courgettes and other summer squashes and tomatoes (which are all technically fruit)
- ❖ Mushrooms
- ❖ Celeriac and Carrots
  - ○ These are both apium and have lower carb counts than other apium family root veg, such as parsnips.

Suboptimal (eat these good for the guts, nutrient dense foods that mostly also have a small carbohydrate load in moderation, with care and enjoyment):

Moderate amounts of
- ❖ Offal (Organ meats)
  - ○ All Offal is excellent for our bodies and enjoying them is part of a healthy life. However, they just slide into suboptimal because they usually carry a small amount of glucose as well as causing a possible vitamin and mineral overload if eaten every day. Once or twice a week at

most is usually enough to get the benefit from these nutritional powerhouses.

- ❖ All soft cheeses, kefir and full fat natural yoghurt
  - ○ These products retain some of the lactose through the manufacturing process but are awesome for your gut heath.
- ❖ Fermented soy products, such as tempeh, natto and miso,
- ❖ Onions, leeks & garlic,
- ❖ All tree nuts such as hazelnuts, almonds, pistachio, brazil, macadamia, pecan
- ❖ Protein based processed foods that have 5 ingredients or less
  - ○ Making it yourself is always better, but not always possible or even practical. This is food such as sausages, hamburgers or part prepared "ready to cook meat with a sauce" type dishes - Read labels, and if there are ingredients in it that you couldn't find to use at home, don't buy it.

Small amounts of

- ❖ Root vegetables rich in colourful phytonutrients such as beetroot, parsnip, and sweet potato,
- ❖ Root spices such as ginger, galangal and turmeric,
- ❖ 70% and over top-quality dark chocolate,
- ❖ Cocoa powder and cocoa nibs,
- ❖ Berry fruit, such as strawberries, raspberries, blueberries and blueberries,

- ❖ Stone fruit, such as peaches, plums, apricots and nectarines
- ❖ Red wine,
- ❖ Stevia (ka'a he'ê)
    - ○ This is an herb that naturally grows in Brazil, Argentina and Paraguay between the Uruguay and Lower Paraguay rivers, widely used by the indigenous Guaraní population for its sweet taste.
    - ○ It as officially "discovered" and given its taxonomy label in the 19th Century by Dr Moises Santiago Bertoni[5].
    - ○ The Guaraní either use it as it is, chew it to sweeten their breath, or dry the herb and crumble to sweeten their food.
    - ○ The Stevia we see in the shops is made by extracting the sweet compounds in the herb, a group of chemicals called "steviol glycosides" - stevioside and rebaudioside A-E. Rebaudioside A being the only one approved for use in the EU at this time.
    - ○ The extract is either dissolved in water and sold as drops (the preferable way to purchase and use) or mixed with a bulking agent to enable it to be "spooned" - sometimes Maltodextrin (a very fluffy form of glucose), but usually the polyol Erythritol, which does have its own issues and is a non-optimal in itself in my opinion.

---

[5] http://www.lowcarbinthe.uk/blog/stevia/

- You only need a tiny amount. Stevia is approximately 200 times sweeter to the tongue than sucrose, however, it can also carry a liquorice aftertaste, and if you use too much it delivers a bitter sensation, rather than a sweet one,
- It can be used for cooking, as it is heat stable to 200 degrees Celsius (392 degrees Fahrenheit)
- It's a suboptimal because using it as you would have used sugar keeps our tongue in the habit of expecting sweet stuff (Yes, your sweet tooth is a habit, more on this in the next part!)

❖ Monk fruit (Luo han guo)

- Monk fruit or "Lo Han" is part of the cucurbitaceae (gourd) family and grows on vines in the southern Chinese Guangxi and Guangdong mountains.[6] The fruit itself tastes rotten soon after it is ripe because it contains high amounts of volatile sulphur-based compounds.
- Historically it was dried and used medicinally as a "lung improver".
- In modern times, the fruit has an antioxidant compound in it that is also intensely sweet - mogroside – which is extracted as a brownish powder and now sold worldwide by China.

---

[6] https://draxe.com/monk-fruit/

- ○ Like Stevia, buying Monk fruit drops is the best way to use this product, as in powdered form it is usually bulked with maltodextrin.
- ○ You only need a tiny amount. Monk Fruit Extract is approximately 150 times sweeter to the tongue than sucrose, however, it can also carry a "off-ish" aftertaste, and just like Stevia, if you use too much it delivers a bitter sensation, rather than a sweet one,
- ○ It is rather expensive, as the Chinese Government do not allow any Monk fruit genetic material to be exported from China, so it can only be grown, harvested and processed in China.
- ○ It can be used for cooking, as it is also heat stable to 200 degrees Celsius (392 degrees Fahrenheit)
- ○ It's a suboptimal for the same reason as Stevia.

Eat in minimal amounts, take extra care.

- ❖ Seeds
  - ○ Sunflower, pumpkin, linseed, hemp, poppy, pine nuts, chia, sesame and cashews.
  - ○ Seeds are nutrient dense, and chia and psyllium especially have nice amounts of soluble fibre.

- However, the "oilseeds" are also high in phytic acid and phytates, as are cashews. Phytic acid can bind with minerals in the gut to prevent absorption. They influence digestive enzymes and also reduce the digestibility of starches, proteins, and fats.

❖ Pulses
  - Such as chickpeas, garden peas and peanuts.
  - Although they are nutrient dense, with nice amounts of fibre and some protein, they pack both a carb punch and also contain high amounts of phytates.
  - Modern cooking practises tend to leave this substance behind, so if you are eating pulses, soaking them for twelve hours, draining and rinsing three times for a total of thirty-six hours and then cooking them at over 65C is a must. Sprouting them and then cooking is also a good way to reduce phytates
  - Pulses represent a protein source that has issues, but they are always better than a non-optimal choice in a pinch, hummus and crudités at a party for instance, or a packet of peanuts grabbed on the run instead of a packet of crisps.

○ If you are a vegetarian, pulses are an "incomplete protein" that is usually paired with rice to create a "complete" protein. In a low carb diet, seeds would be a better choice, but please do your own research here, as I'm not a vegetarian.

Non-Optimal (really not at all good for the body. Enjoyed without guilt once in a blue moon, if at all):

Avoid eating
- ❖ All potatoes except sweet.
- ❖ All grain and grain products, especially wheat; pasta, rice, bread, rusks, cake, biscuits, crackers, cereal bars, as well as sweet corn, oats, spelt, barley, quinoa etc.
  - ○ Apart from their high carb load, grains also have high levels of phytates.
- ❖ All unfermented soy products; Edamame, Tofu, commercial soya milk,
  - ○ Raw Soya contains phytates, goitrogens and phytoestrogens. Fermentation removes these harmful compounds.[7]
- ❖ All highly processed food products.
- ❖ All processed low-fat products.

---

[7]http://probiotics.mercola.com/fermented-vs-unfermented-soy.html

- ❖ All plant-based oils from seeds; sunflower, safflower, corn, vegetable
  - ○ Seed oils contain high levels of Omega 6 fatty acids, and eating more of these than the Omega 3 fatty acids contributes to cell aging. As it is harder to eat more Omega 3 than to remove Omega 6 fatty acids if seed oils are included as a major fat source in the diet, these are non-optimal for that reason, even though they contain zero grams of carbohydrate.
- ❖ All tropical and autumn fruit.
  - ○ Such as grapes, banana, apples, pears, mangoes and pineapple
- ❖ All forms of sugar; granulated, honey, agave syrup, maple syrup.
  - ○ Anything ending in -ose[8].
- ❖ Alcohol
  - ○ I'm not saying never, heck, I enjoy a nice glass of suboptimal gut microbiome enhancing red wine from time to time, but overall, Alcohol is damaging to the body and contributes nothing but body fat in the visceral area. I'll talk about this in excruciating details later

---

Remove

❖ Any form of fibreless fruit product; Juice, fruit leathers, apple sauce, jam & jellies.

○ Fruit is made by nature with fibre, and fibre buffers the fructose within fruit to render it less harmful.

❖ All synthetic trans-fats, such as margarine and partially hydrogenated vegetable oil from your diet.

○ These fats are not found at all in nature and our bodies are simply not equipped to deal with them. They contribute to accelerated cell breakdown and to coronary heart disease (CHD) and so are at the very bottom of the non-optimal end of the scale, even though they also have zero grams of carbohydrate! [9]

❖ Artificial Sweeteners, especially aspartame

○ There are studies that show that artificial sweeteners can increase hunger by stimulating Insulin and so cause us to eat more to compensate, so ultimately, we are aiming to remove them from out diet. Although they are useful at the beginning of your low carb journey, only use them to get over the initial bump, and then I strongly advise that you aim to ramp down until you have removed them entirely from your diet.

---

[9] https://www.theguardian.com/society/2006/sep/27/health.food

- As I said above with Stevia, use of sweeteners keeps you in the habit of a sweet tooth[10]
- ❖ Polyol based sweetener products
  - These naturally occurring very long chain carbohydrates taste sweet, perform the same chemistry in baking as sugar does but are like fibre, in that they are almost indigestible to the body.
  - I say almost, as some of the shorter chains of the family, sorbitol, mannitol and maltitol are up to 60% digested into glucose, and as such act like "half-hit" carbohydrates to our systems. Even the longer chain ones, xylitol and erythritol are still around 15-20% digestible, and all this really adds up to bad news for both us and our guts as they tend to ferment on their way through our bowels, killing off our gut flora.
  - Consuming too much polyol leads to bloating, farting and potentially cramping and a sharp run to the toilet with violent diarrhoea. This effect is known as "The polywobbles".

---

[10] Yang Q. Gain weight by "going diet?" Artificial sweeteners and the neurobiology of sugar cravings: Neuroscience 2010. The Yale Journal of Biology and Medicine-2010;83(2):101-108.
https://www.ncbi.nlm.nih.gov/pmc/articles/PMC2892765/

- If you ever read the reviews on Amazon for sugar-free gummi bears, you will know exactly what I'm talking about![11]

○ All polyols work as laxatives by drawing water into the large intestine when they are poorly absorbed, which moves the food quickly through the intestines, triggering bowel movements. The shorter chain polyols are more likely to cause this effect than the longer ones.

- This is exactly why prunes are laxative, as well as a healthy amount of fibre, they contain relatively large amounts of Sorbitol compared to other fruit.

○ Whilst polyols occur in small amounts naturally in vegetables and fruit, and whilst inside a food they don't usually cause any issues for most people, they are an IBS trigger.

○ If you are going low carb to help your IBS, (which it usually very much does), know that Polyols are a "Fermentable Oligosaccharides, Disaccharides, Monosaccharides and Polyols" (FODMAP) and so to be strictly avoided[12].

---

[11]https://www.buzzfeed.com/michaelrusch/haribo-gummy-bear-reviews-on-amazon-are-the-most-insane-thin

[12]https://www.alittlebityummy.com/blog/what-are-polyols/

- o Xylitol is deathly toxic to dogs.
- o Erythritol is a potent insecticide.

I call this overall way of looking at food the OSN scale, mostly because it's way quicker to type than "optimal, suboptimal, non-optimal"!

I appreciate that the above is a great deal to take in, so to help out, the list without the explanations is in the printables supplement, and I've also made a helpful graphic that covers most of the above in a single place:

I've also posted this as a webpage with a colour graphic here, so that you can have a handy reference both for yourself and to show others:

http://www.lowcarbinthe.uk/osnscale/

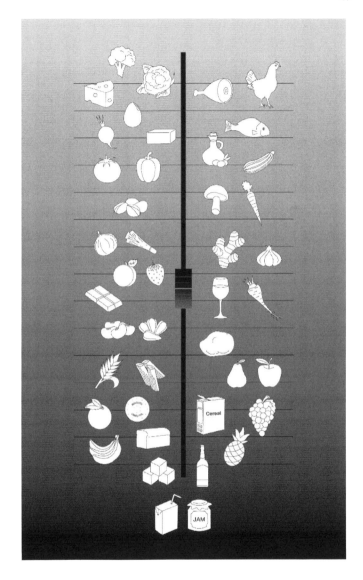

Naturally, these lists are not exhaustive, there is simply too much food to classify! So, use the OSN scale and your discernment to classify your food.

1) How many carbs does it have?
   0-5g - optimal
   6-10g - If a vegetable, optimal.
   If not a vegetable, suboptimal
   Over 10g - suboptimal,
   Over 25g - non-optimal.

2) How nutrient dense is it?
   Nutrient dense - bumps it up the scale
   Nutrient sparse - slides it down the scale

3) How much harm it does the body
   Little to none - bumps it up the scale
   Very harmful indeed - slides it down to non-optimal

So, look at the nutrient density, "human food suitability" and how much good it will do the body versus the carbohydrate load the food carries and how processed it is.

You will notice that there are no "banned / forbidden / naughty / sinful" foods in this world view; assigning negativity to food is simply setting yourself up for guilt and failure. Which is not at all productive for a happy life.

This is where living by the third tenet (*Make every mouthful as optimal as possible, given the circumstances in which you find yourself in*) comes into play; aim to make choices of optimal foods mostly and the suboptimal ones occasionally.

Take it one mouthful at a time, and as you go along, listen to what your body is asking you for, it knows what it wants and will ask you for it once you get rid of all the processed junk.

We are going to be working on that more in part two of the book, but for now, simply keep in mind that the pareto principle (AKA the 80/20 rule)[13] applies to food as well as project management!

---

[13] https://en.wikipedia.org/wiki/Pareto_principle

The nine shifts to a low carb way of eating[14]

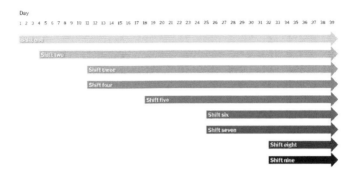

Unlike most "diet plans," I'm not looking to give you "a quick win" on the weighing scale. This is because how much we weigh does not equate in any way to how much body fat we are carrying around - Our weight is the weight of our whole body and its contents: fat, muscles, bone, viscera, blood, hormones, lipids, glucose, glycogen, water & the content of our stomach, bowels & bladder.

When you begin any diet, but especially a low carb one where you cut carbs sharply and immediately, most people usually see a quick drop of around 3Kg (7lbs) on the scale - this is our body using up its glycogen stores. Seeing a drop on the scale gives us a good feeling, because we have been programmed that "weight" is the be all and end all, but this quick result has virtually

---

[14] Colour graphic and shift headings here:
http://www.lowcarbinthe.uk/nine-shifts/

nothing to do with burning off our fat stores and returning us to optimum.

Our bodies then act to balance what's going on, which means that most people then maybe see a 1kg (~2.2lbs) maximum drop the next week followed nothing at all the week after that. Which is where, if you are scale fixated, you can get somewhat depressed and disheartened.

Meanwhile, when you are eating in a low carb manner, your body is recomposing. Fat is being burned whilst muscle and bone density are being regained. These two factors cancel each other out on the scale, but they mean that your body is getting smaller, more dense and healthier. Which is a much better way of looking at it!

When weight is literally the worst measure we can choose to measure progress, why are we emotionally tied to the weighing scales? Because that's the way our society as well as the diet and medical industries is set up - weight has been the measure of a person since before the common era.

We are educated to value this measure beyond all others, even though logically, it is nonsensical to do so. Our body weight varies massively on a day-to-day basis. We can weigh one thing in the morning and easily be a kilo or two heavier or lighter at bedtime.

So, I'm going to ask you to use a tape measure at a minimum of every two weeks and judge your progress by how your clothes are fitting (& buying new ones as your size reduces!)

Why am I asking you to do this? Because people look at us and make a judgment on how big or small we are, and then convert that in their head linguistically to "weight" as an equivalence of fat.

But as none of us carry our weight number around in our aura above our heads as a neon sign, why is "weight" a judge of our size or our health?!

Your size, shape and body composition are more consistent measures of fat burning and muscle and bone restoration, and this awareness of your body both starts opening communication lines with it and allows you to feel it becoming more and more optimal.

I'd say that this way of looking at things is way more exciting than being trapped in the mental judgement of a number on a weighing scale. Being involved in our body is a good thing, as it's an important part of us.

I'm realistic enough however to know that you are still going to weigh yourself. Hey, I still weigh myself occasionally! The scale habit is a hard one to drop, however, I'm simply asking you to put little to no value in the result of weighing yourself as any form of indicator of your progress. All the feelings that the number on the scale give you are really really unhelpful as we progress into a low carb way of life.

As you move through the shifts you will be mentally battling with the training we all receive, that food is the enemy and your body is a weak-willed traitor for wanting it. We are taught that if we only have some discipline, we can become thin.

Which is why I've set up the system so that your shift to a low carb way of eating happens gracefully over a short time period. I designed the shifts in such a way to help you recognise that "weight loss" messaging is deeply flawed and to support you through changing your diet, as well as subtly working on your mindset and your habits before we start digging in deep during part two.

I recommend that you proceed in this manner: complete shift one, then follow a "no more than 7 days" dictum for the other steps, flowing directly through steps 3, 6 and 8 as directed.

At this pace, it will take you a maximum of 39 days to fully complete the shifts, which is how I have written it below. Taking the next five weeks to build & embed new habits along the way eases you, your mind and your body into a low carb life.

Here's the graphic again to help you understand the flow:

Five weeks??? You must be joking! What if I just want to get on with it now?

The first shift takes a **non-negotiable** three days. We are working on a new paradigm here, and you need the self-knowledge and realisation that shift one gives to stand any chance of keeping your optimal body once you achieve it. Taking these three days to do self-discovery is honouring and serving your mind, your body and yourself.

The first three days are a little bit of a conscious mindset shifting, which paves the way for bigger changes later – Martin Gabel said "*Don't just do something, stand there*" and this is what you are doing for these three days.

Many of us go through life mindlessly, and "always keeping busy" has become a badge of honour. What that means is that usually food and self-care become one of our lowest priorities.

So, this three-day analysis allows us to start the process of reconnecting with ourselves, it's a step towards "mind, body, spirit" not being at constant war.

However, once you have completed the first shift, you can progress through the rest of the food shifts at the pace you desire within the "no more than 7 days" dictum, and shifts 3, 6 and 8 need no pauses anyway.

If you are a "go for it" person, there is no harm at all in jumping right in and proceeding through each food shift at speed.

Complete the first shift and then do the next eight all at once and be eating in a low-carb manner from the 4th day. Or, you could choose to make one (or two) food shifts every day until you have swapped over in about a week.

NB: Swapping over to a low carb way of eating all at once may well lead to "keto-flu" as the body takes about a week to fully adapt, and protests loudly to you whilst it does so. There is a note on what "keto-flu" is and how to avoid this in shift 5.

However, if you work slightly more slowly and wean yourself off your current eating patterns and into a healthier relationship with yourself and the food you eat, I believe that you will gain better long terms results.

Shift 1, Day 1: Make a three-day non-judgemental qualitative food diary

We are going to start our journey with some fact gathering - knowledge is power.

I would like you to get yourself a journal; take your arm, chest, waist, tummy, hip and thigh measurements (and yes, if you must, your weight) and for the first three days of the journey keep a food diary. This is not a calorie or quantity diary, it's a food quality diary.

If you need a little guidance as to how to lay this out, I've made some sample pages for the printables supplement. To remind you, the details on how you get this are at the end of the book.

As I said, this first shift is non-negotiable. You could skip it but taking these three days to learn about where you are now will benefit you as you learn about yourself. It will also make it easier longer term, as you will be able to pick up themes in your current eating patterns, and so have more ability to avoid your obvious pitfalls.

Doing this exercise will help you know how big a life change this will be for you, as well as hopefully pointing out those foods that may well have way more emotions attached to them than is healthy, and where you will need to do some work once we get into working on our how we think and feel about food.

Please make notes on:

- How much whole food you eat vs. how much processed food?
- How many meals you cook from real ingredients vs. ready-meals and/or low-calorie, sugar loaded products that you buy and ding in 5 minutes?
- How much care you take over both preparing and eating your meals and snacks?
- How much snacking you do day-to-day?
- How much food ends up randomly in your mouth and when?
  - This shows you your "mindless eating" patterns
- What times of the day you eat. Is this around the same time every day, or rather random?
- How much fluid (tea, coffee, water, fizzy drinks, alcohol) you consume?
- Finally, and most importantly, note any and all feelings you have around the food you are consuming.
  - Writing this will help you to see where you have negative emotions to deal with, as well as the food itself.

I would advise you to continue journaling, as it will support you through the journey.

If you can see where you are coming from and can be honest with yourself about where you are going in terms of both food and feelings, this will make shifting our thinking towards mindfulness and success far easier to achieve.

If there is no change in the way that we think about food, there is a statistically much higher chance of regaining the fat that you drop - via any intervention, not just a low carb way of eating.[15]

Using the information you find out from journaling, I also strongly recommend that you do a Forgiveness Exercise around any feeling that have come up for you: http://tiny.cc/forgivenessexercise

If you are here with me now, then I'm pretty sure that, just like I did, you are very likely to have a broken relationship with food that has been brought about by how you've been taught to view food and your body in the past.

---

[15] http://www.mindfuleatinghk.com/resources/research-articles

It also helps to have people to talk to along the way, people that get where you are now and can help you out,

Joining my Low Carb in the UK Facebook group: http://tiny.cc/LCUKFBG is a fantastic way to get support.

I hang out in there regularly, as well as over 6000 people (as at publishing date) that are all living a happy low carb life.

Shift 2, Day 4: Avoid obvious "excess sugar" foods

On day four, start to avoid obvious excess sugars in prepared sweet foods – such as sweets, chocolate, biscuits, cakes, sweet pastries, ice cream and other desserts.

Look at your diary and work on either dropping one of these sugary food types a day at a time, or cut them all out in one go, which ever you feel is easiest for you. Don't replace these foods and don't worry about avoiding excess sugar in processed savoury foods or drinks right now - this comes a little later.

Aim to be "mostly obvious sugar avoiding" within a week of starting out (by day 11 at the latest) - however, for this shift, the sooner you shift the better. The longer you take here, the more likely you will not progress on and return to eating sweets again.

Start thinking about making choices of food that are nutrient dense, but don't worry too much about this as yet, as that's our next shift. As you are still eating sugars and starches, your hunger signals will still be not optimally tuned yet but start to observe them anyway.

Finally start to focus on food quality and start work to maintain the three tenets.

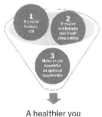

A healthier you

Shift 3, Day 11: Focus on food quality and "eating naturally"

Begin to really focus on food quality and eating foods that you can make from scratch - the food we eat creates our body; if you eat rubbish foods, you will have a rubbish body.

Start looking at the ingredient list of food labels - if a product has "weird sounding" ingredients in it, (i.e. you could not create the dish in your own kitchen) do not buy that product.

Start to emphasise choosing optimal foods (proteins, fats and leafy greens) in your meals and snacks and choose to add more of the more suboptimal colourful vegetables with meals.

Eat to satisfy your hunger and begin to form the habit of thinking about nutrient density. Even if the food you choose at this stage is a carb laden one, start to avoid the obviously processed ones, the ones that are stripped of their natural fibre and nutrients.

Move straight on to shift 4 - this shift of viewing and choosing food and eating using a qualitative lens is all about habit forming.

Making new habits around food and maintaining the three tenets is key to success and future wellness, so I'm going to be repeating myself on this point quite a bit.

Shift 4, Day 11: Avoid wheat and wheat containing products & do not replace avoided wheat with other starchy carbohydrates or "gluten free" products

You are already avoiding cakes, sweet pastries and biscuits, but with this shift, start to avoid all wheat products as much as possible. Wheat foods such as bread, pasta, & savoury pastries are the main targets in this shift, but there are plenty of pre-prepared foods that have wheat flour added to them. Reading the labels will show you the wheat content of a food.

This is our first serious challenge - UK Culture is very bread centred and most "on-the-run" options are based around sandwiches, and we use wheat flour to thicken and bulk a multitude of processed food.

Why avoid wheat specifically at this stage but not other grains?

The wheat protein complex in modern gluten contains a protein called gliadin. Unlike all other proteins, this one directly stimulates appetite and induces cravings to eat more of it. [16]

---

[16]Wheat Belly by William Davis MD
- http://amzn.to/2CdYNNG

Wheat is not the only gluten containing grain, but it is the grain that is most prevalent in the western diet and so our most plentiful source of gliadin.

NB: Do not replace wheat products with manufactured "gluten-free" food equivalents - these contain other starches that scores higher on the glycaemic index (and so cause more hunger) than wheat does.

During this shift, eat rice, oats, rye, corn and other non-wheat grains as you did previously - we will begin to avoid them shortly however, so do not get into a habit of replacing wheat with another starchy carbohydrate.

Aim to be wheat avoiding as soon as you can, again within a maximum of 7 days of starting this shift.

As always, focus on food quality and maintain the three tenets.

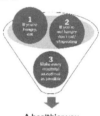

A healthier you

Shift 5, Day 18: Increase quantity of water consumed, balance electrolytes and avoid drinking your sugar

Start drinking plain water if you do not already do so. This can be difficult for some people, because water can be boring! Tea and coffee are ok, and green tea especially has a large amount of gut microbiome supporting compounds in it, but water is better in terms of body function.

Drinking water and non-caffeinated fluids massively assists liver and kidney function, which helps the body to burn its fat stores away efficiently. Having an "always full" glass or bottle of water nearby and sipping from it is the good habit we are building in this shift. Don't worry about how much right now, simply start to build the habit.

Add a splash of lemon or lime juice to water and tea as you can (it would taste so weird in coffee!), this helps promote good pH balance.

A note on milk here: Although milk is nutritious, it also contains generous amounts of the natural sugar lactose. If you drink your tea and coffee white, that splash of milk can add up fast to an excess of lactose. Cream has the same nutrient values but way less lactose, so use cream in the place of milk where you can.

Another habit to get into is adding in a mug of good quality bullion, broth or stock into your daily liquid intake. This helps to balance your electrolytes which enhances overall well-being and also supports fat burning.

NB: If you are speeding through the shifts, increasing electrolytes[17] by drinking some good quality bone broth and using Himalayan (pink) salt on food or taking a specific electrolyte zero sugar sports drink (https://amzn.to/2q33XIf) combats the symptoms of "Keto-flu" http://tiny.cc/ketoflu

Dr Ken Barry and his wife Neisha invented "Ketorade" - A good DIY way to replenish electrolytes, to stave off the keto flu symptoms as well as being an all round good thing to drink most if not every day. https://youtu.be/_EftSmV4UMU

---

[17] https://draxe.com/electrolyte-imbalance/

"Ketorade"

In a glass litre container:

- ❖ Juice from ½ lime or lemon
- ❖ 2 tablespoons of Apple Cider Vinegar "with the mother" (ACV)
  - ○ "The mother" is a cloudy substance floating in some bottles of vinegar. It is the substance that causes vinegar to sour and is believed to be rich in health-boosting natural protein and healthy bacteria.[18]
- ❖ ½ tsp of Lo-salt (K based table condiment)
- ❖ ½ tsp of unprocessed salt (pink, grey, black, sea, rock)
- ❖ 5-10 drops of liquid Stevia extract (to taste)
- ❖ Add a dropperful of liquid Mg if you are having muscle spasms, constipation, or trouble sleeping
- ❖ 1ltr of a good quality sparkling mineral water
  - ○ Use one which has a more or less equal amount of calcium (Ca) and magnesium (Mg). Many mineral waters have a dominance of Ca, which throws Mg levels out of whack in the body
- ❖ 1 drop of an edible high-quality orange, lemon or lime essential oil, to mask the ACV smell if required (this is why we use glass, as essential oils eat plastics)

---

[18]https://www.hollandandbarrett.com/the-health-hub/5-benefits-of-apple-cider-vinegar-with-the-mother/

Tweak the amount of Stevia and lime/lemon to make your "Ketorade" taste the best to you. Make it up the night before, bung it in the fridge and done.

Finally, start to avoid sugar-loaded beverages (e.g. soft drinks and fruit juices) from your liquid consumption and stop adding sugar to any beverage consumed.

Use "diet drinks" and artificial sweeteners at this stage to help if you need them and aim to ramp down use over time. "Ketorade" can also very much hit the "missing fizzy drinks spot" as well as being actively good for the body, unlike the fizzy drinks it is replacing!

Aim to have removed liquid sugars from your diet within a maximum of 7 days. Increasing water intake is an ongoing piece, adding around 2 litres of pure water to your fluid intake over time is a good thing.

As always, focus on your food quality and maintain the three tenets.

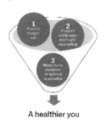

A healthier you

If you are geeky, use this table to work out how much water is optimal for your body:

Weight (lb)	Weight (kg)	Water (ltr)
290 lb	131 kg	4.83 ltr
280 lb	127 kg	4.55 ltr
270 lb	122 kg	4.27 ltr
260 lb	117 kg	3.98 ltr
250 lb	113 kg	3.70 ltr
240 lb	108 kg	3.41 ltr
220 lb	99 kg	3.13 ltr
200 lb	91 kg	2.98 ltr
180 lb	82 kg	2.55 ltr
160 lb	73 kg	2.27 ltr
140 lb	64 kg	1.98 ltr
120 lb	54 kg	1.70 ltr
100 lb	45 kg	1.41 ltr
80 lb	36 kg	1.13 ltr

Remember that you will need to drink more water if you're physically active and when it is warm.

Shift 6, Day 25: Ensure that you are eating good amounts of fat and protein

Now that you are avoiding most obvious processed carbohydrate-based foods, check in with yourself and ensure that you have increased your levels of fat and protein to meet your hunger levels, as we set out in shift 3.

Maintain the three tenets, especially the first one - If you are hungry, eat! Choose something optimal and chow down to satisfy your hunger. This will stop you and your body feeling deprivation as you have removed it's usually sources of energy by reducing the starches and sugars. Don't fall into the trap that hunger is a good thing, right now, it isn't, and you have no need to feel it at all.

Also, it's easy to cook low-carb meals that are appetising and nutritious; Fat and Protein containing foods, combined with vegetables are very tasty. One of the reasons that our prepared foods are so sugar laden is that when you remove fat, you remove taste - which the food industry adds back in by adding sugar to the product.

If you need to snack, make choices from fatty protein foods, such as a piece of cheese, a couple of slices of ham, some sugar-free gelatine jelly with some cream or a handful of nuts.

It's at this point that we are starting to subconsciously work on the way we think and feel about food (I'm sneaky like that!) as changing your diet is as much about our what our mind is up to as it is about doing it, and if you feel deprivation, you are far more likely to not make a change.

Also, having abundant and plentiful nutritious food sends the signal to your body that it's ok to burn off its stored fat. There is no need to hoard when food is plentiful, and your body needs to be reassured on that point. After all, it has no sense of time, it works in the now.

This is one reason why low-calorie diets cause issues, as when calories are restricted, the body ramps down energy requirements as it has no idea how long the famine will last. This is the main reason why a low-calorie diet feels so tiring and also a touch depressing, as anything that reduces energy output is a depressant.

As we are now avoiding the majority of the body's usually preferred energy source, glucose, the body initially sees itself as having less energy available and so it ramps down energy consumption. However, as it sees that overall food intake is good, and that there is a nice amount of the secondary energy source in our food, AKA fat, it knows that energy is plentiful.

So, in a few days, it swaps over to using our secondary energy source as a preference and starts to burn energy happily, and also more enthusiastically than before!

Which is important to know as we head into shift 7 and start avoiding more glucose sources!

Move straight on to shift 7 - this shift is reinforcing shift 3, as well as ensuring that we are eating to hunger from optimal fatty protein choices when we are hungry, as well as viewing and choosing food and eating using a qualitative lens is all about habit forming.

Shift 7, Day 25: Avoid processed carbs

Start to avoid overly-processed foods that contain refined sugars and starches - typically products that are aimed at the low-fat diet market and pre-packaged "junk" foods.

You've been reading labels anyway, to check for obvious wheat and sugar, but now, start to pay attention to the "Nutrition Information per 100g" on the food label.

Nutrition

Typical Values	100g Contains	Each slice (typically 44g) contains	% RI *	RI* for an average adult
Energy	985kJ 235kcal	435kJ 105kcal	5%	8400kJ 2000kcal
Fat	1.5g	0.7g	1%	70g
of which saturates	0.3g	0.1g	1%	20g
Carbohydrate	45.5g	20.g		
of which sugars	3.8g	1.7g	2%	90g
Fibre	2.8g	1.2g		
Protein	7.7g	3.4g		
Salt	1.0g	0.4g	7%	6g

This pack contains 16 servings

*Reference intake of an average adult (8400kJ / 2000kcal)

A typical UK Nutrition information panel
(This label is from Bread, a non-optimal food)

As a rule of thumb,

❖ Any food that is not a vegetable and has more than 5g of carbohydrate per 100g is usually a suboptimal food.

❖ Any food that has more than 25g of carbohydrate per 100g is usually a non-optimal food

○ NB: There are some natural foods that have more than 25g per 100g, such as garlic. These fall into the suboptimal range of the scale because they pack such a nutrient punch that they are worth the carbohydrate load in small amounts.

Some foods however will always be non-optimal, despite having a low carb count. This is because their carbs are coming from non-optimal sources (such as "protein rolls", these contain wheat, soy, sugar and no real nutrition), or they contain ingredients that are unnatural, such as polyols, vegetable oils, sweeteners or trans fats. Most low carb substitute products fall under this category.

As this habit beds in further, from a finesse point of view, starchy foods are more optimal than sugary foods. This is because sucrose becomes glucose and fructose in the body, whereas starch turns into only glucose. I'll talk more about this in the science section.

Do use your common sense when choosing food. If you only need to use a spoonful of the food stuff (such as when adding ketchup or a tsp of nut butter for snacking)

then do so. You are not adding a massive carb load if you are only using a tiny amount of that food or condiment.

For instance, if you need a touch of tomato ketchup with your eggs to enjoy them, then have some.

Yes, ketchup has sugar, but you don't eat 100g at a time. Also, the lycopene in the cooked tomatoes is a fabulous antioxidant, especially if you have a male body. Buy a "low sugar, low salt" ketchup, or make some yourself and enjoy it.

Shift 8, Day 32: Drink alcohol only in moderation, if at all

Alcohol impairs judgement and hijacks digestion - The body sees it as a poison and acts to remove it from the body ASAP - this means that the liver processes it for energy and simply stores all other calories consumed along with it. Alcohol also stops fat burning dead in its tracks until all alcohol has been burned out of the system, whilst also causing damage to the liver as it is processed.

As optimal liver health is a major concern whilst your body is growing slimmer and healthier, aim to drastically reduce alcohol intake to 3-5 units per week at most. If you want your body to ditch fat faster, remove it from your diet totally.

A low-carb way of eating lowers alcohol tolerance. Most people find that a glass or two at most makes them very tipsy indeed.

Finally, if you have been drinking, be very conscious that the first tenet doesn't apply fully when we are intoxicated - alcohol causes false hunger.

Alcohol stimulates the production of Ghrelin, the appetite Stimulating hormone (I'll talk more about the actions of our hormones in the science section)

This means that you are far more likely to be hungry when drinking alcohol and then as inhibition is lowered, and until habits are reformed, far more likely to choose salty, carb-containing snacks, that will possibly seem "not too bad" as judgement is also impaired.

In terms of what to drink, certain types of alcoholic beverage that are more detrimental than others:

- ❖ Spirits are sugar free and so are the preferential choice if you are drinking alcohol.
    - o Obviously, only choose sugar-free mixers, or drink them neat.
- ❖ A glass of sparkling wine is the best wine choice, followed by dry reds and then white wines.
    - o Obviously, sweet wines contain larger amounts of sugar per glass than dry wines.
- ❖ Avoid all forms of beer - It is liquid bread so contains gluten. It also phytoestrogen compounds that promote visceral fat storage (the "beer-belly").
    - o If you desperately want a beer, Pilsner type are the way to go, as most of the sugar has turned to alcohol.
- ❖ Avoid all liqueurs - they are chock full of sugar.

Like shifts 3 and 6, there is no need to wait to proceed to shift 9 - Avoiding alcohol is an on-going process, and I believe is a key to success and future wellness.

Shift 9, day 32: Avoid natural carbohydrate foods

Just because something is natural doesn't mean that it is good for the body. Arsenic and Cyanide being two natural substances that illustrate this perfectly!

In this final shift, we are at the point where we are choosing to avoid and reduce consumption of foods that are naturally high in carbohydrate and are nutrient sparse, or have more sugar than other nutrients inside them:

Start to avoid non-optimal, naturally high carb food:
- ❖ Honey, Agave, Date Sugar, Palm sugar, Coconut sugar and all other forms of "natural" sugar
  - ○ There are more than 50 names for sugar used by the food industry, some of which sound natural and harmless, so be aware[19]
- ❖ All high-starch cereal grains (Rice, Oats, Rye, Corn etc)
- ❖ All high-starch root vegetables - potatoes, yams, cassava and most other tubers.
  - ○ (There are a few that are suboptimal rather than non-optimal - I list those in the next section)
- ❖ All high-sugar tropical fruits (i.e. Oranges, Grapefruit, Bananas, Papaya, Mango, Pineapple

---

[19]https://www.bhf.org.uk/heart-matters-magazine/nutrition/sugar-salt-and-fat/names-for-sugar-infographic/different-names-for-sugar

etc), and high-sugar Autumn fruits (Apples, Pears, Quince, Meddlers etc)

Avoiding some of these foods, especially fruit may give you feelings. We are told that all fruit is fantastic for us, however, the higher sugar fruit is nowhere near as nutrient loaded as vegetables. For instance, gram for gram there is way more vitamin C in broccoli and strawberries than there is in oranges. Most tropical fruit are low in antioxidants compared to berry and stone fruit.

We are also told that fructose is less harmful to us than sugar. It isn't.

Fructose is nature's way of making us fat for winter. It is converted directly into body fat by the liver and doesn't stimulate Insulin to do so. I'll dig deeply into why fructose, especially fructose delivered without fibre is one of the most harmful things that we can put into our body which is not instantly poisonous in the science section.

As well as avoiding the non -optimal high carb foods, we are also reducing consumption of the below suboptimal foods but ensuring that they are still in our diet - these are carb loaded choices that are also nutrient-dense and antioxidant filled and so they are worth their carbohydrate load to us to enjoy in moderate to small amounts:

- Legumes (peas, peanuts, lentils, chickpeas, beans etc)
- Colourful root vegetables such as sweet potatoes, parsnips, carrots and beetroot
- Squashes such as butternut squash and pumpkin
- Onion, garlic and leeks
- Dark Chocolate
  - I advise that if you are going to eat chocolate ensure that it is a high percentage cocoa solids chocolate. At least 70%, 85% for preference.
  - Cocoa mass is packed heart healthy fats, antioxidants and flavonoids and also has a fair whack of Magnesium (~146mg per 100g) as well.
  - Ensure that what you buy is a quality chocolate, as properly handled cocoa solids are excellent for the body.
  - Avoid chocolate that is cheap, sugar filled, made with polyols and/or has other fats in it bar cocoa butter.
    Adding vegetable oil to chocolate removes the heart healthy fats
    Mass production of cheap chocolate renders it virtually nutrient barren.
  - Lots of sugar, or polyols rather than sugar simply lowers the amount of cocoa mass available to us
  - If you add milk to chocolate it binds the flavonoids making them biologically unavailable to us.
  - That and life is simply too short to eat cheap crappy chocolate!

- ❖ Berry fruit and stone fruit (strawberries, raspberries, peaches, plums, apricots etc)
    - ○ Here is an article I wrote back in 2003 about fruit if you want to learn more: http://tiny.cc/lcfruitchoices

Day 39: Congratulations! You are now living a low-carb life!

That's it. You've shifted your diet over to a low carb way of eating and started to think about food in a whole new light as well as beginning to embed some great habits along the way.

All there is to it now is maintaining your focus on food quality and the three tenets.

I know, I make it sound so easy! Honestly though, as you keep on keeping on eating food that has a more optimal value for your body, the desire to eat food that makes us feel rubbish diminishes and so it is much easier to maintain the habit of eating optimal food over time

How to plan your low carb day

If you want to get in deep with weekly and monthly menu planning, I've written a very short book on this already: Control your Low Carb week http://amzn.to/2hgdcBT

To get you started though, here's a few meal ideas. Mix and match as you wish, recipes where required are either linked or in the printables supplement. (Details of how to get this on the last page of the book.)

This selection is just for inspiration – never be afraid to mix it up, eat a breakfast for lunch, or a dinner for breakfast! Approach food with curiosity and playfulness, try stuff out, find what you like and enjoy what you eat!

Breakfasts

- ❖ Leftovers from the night before (never underestimate the usefulness of this!)
- ❖ "Monica's Muesli" with yoghurt, Coyo or cream
- ❖ Bullet proof coffee
- ❖ Breakfast sausage muffins
- ❖ Greek full fat yoghurt and
  - o a few berries or one diced dried apricot
  - o 50g toasted flaked almond and a few berries
- ❖ Scrambled eggs with cheese, cheese and ham, salmon or spinach
- ❖ Scotch egg
- ❖ Two large boiled/fried/poached eggs with a few of rashers of crispy streaky bacon/turkey bacon

or two premium sausages and sautéed mushrooms

❖ Omelette
  ○ Bacon, spinach and cheese
  ○ Spanish-ish – diced pepper and onion with some cooked radish cubes
  ○ Ham and Mushroom
  ○ Whatever you fancy putting in it!
❖ Sliced avocado and Parma ham or crispy bacon
❖ Baked eggs in avocado
❖ Two boiled eggs, avocado, chopped spinach, a little chilli and a dash of lemon juice all mashed together
❖ Bacon sandwich made with low carb "bread"[20]
❖ Eggs Royal/Florentine/Benedict with a toasted almond & coconut flour "English muffin"
❖ Fried halloumi with egg, mushrooms, tomatoes
❖ "Porridge"/ "NOatmeal"
❖ Kippers with a dot of melted butter and some wilted spinach
❖ Smoked salmon and cream cheese on "cloud bread"
❖ 2 Mozzarella balls
❖ 100g packet of macadamia, pecan, hazel or brazil nuts
❖ 120g pack of ham
❖ Lump of cheese

---

[20]http://www.thelondoner.me/2014/03/mums-low-carb-bread.html gets really good reviews! Ensure that the flax meal (AKA ground linseed) is very fresh, or it will taste fishy and horrid – Linseeds go rancid very easily, so grind them yourself and then keep any excess in the freezer

- ❖ 300g pot of full-fat cottage cheese
- ❖ A creamy protein shake
- ❖ Nut butter, either straight from the jar or spread on a slice of toasted low carb "bread"

Lunches

- ❖ Scotch egg meatloaf slices with a salad
- ❖ Scrambled egg, smoked salmon and an "English muffin"
- ❖ Smoked mackerel pate with celery and radishes
- ❖ A herb omelette made with 3 eggs and a tablespoon of full fat soft cheese
- ❖ 3 premium brand sausages with spinach and salad greens
- ❖ Broccoli cheese soup with a side of ham https://www.wholesomeyum.com/recipes/brocc oli-cheese-soup-low-carb-gluten-free/
- ❖ Cheese wrapped in ham slices
- ❖ Chicken avocado salad
- ❖ Griddled halloumi with salad & extra virgin olive oil
- ❖ Omelette
  - o Bacon, spinach and cheese
  - o Spanish-ish – diced pepper and onion with some cooked radish cubes
  - o Ham and Mushroom
  - o Whatever you fancy putting in it!
- ❖ Romaine lettuce "cups" with tuna mayonnaise, sliced cucumber and diced spring onion
- ❖ Avocado, tomato and onion and feta cheese mixed up with cauliflower "cous cous"
- ❖ Green salad with olives and avocados

- ❖ Chicken and vegetable broth with a spoonful of almond butter afterwards

Dinners

- ❖ Steak in Dijon mustard cream sauce, with mushrooms, purple sprouting broccoli, sliced red peppers and green beans. http://emerils.com/126904/dijon-mustard-cream-sauce
- ❖ Steak with sautéed mushrooms & melted blue cheese with a side of salad
- ❖ Paneer and spinach curry and cauli rice
- ❖ Bratwurst with sauerkraut and cauliflower cheese
- ❖ Bolognaise sauce with mushrooms, on courgetti or boodles
- ❖ Cauliflower pizza with toppings of your choice and salad
- ❖ Fathead pizza with toppings of your choice and salad
- ❖ Pan fried salmon fillet with fried cabbage and leek
- ❖ "Southern Fried chicken" and coleslaw https://ketogasm.com/keto-fried-chicken-recipe-baked-oven/
- ❖ Pork belly with courgette and cabbage or green beans
- ❖ Pork chop, asparagus, Brussels sprouts with cheese sauce http://tiny.cc/cheesesauce
- ❖ Pork chop in a creamy mushroom sauce with crispy fried kale

- ❖ Slow cooker beef chilli with full fat sour cream, salad, and low carb tortillas https://recipes.sainsburys.co.uk/recipes/main-courses/slow-cooker-beef-chilli (minus kidney beans!) https://www.ketoconnect.net/recipe/low-carb-tortillas/
- ❖ Vegetable curry with cauliflower rice
- ❖ Pulled pork with swede mash and green beans https://www.ibreatheimhungry.com/slow-cooker-pulled-pork-low-carb-gluten-free
- ❖ Baked cod, oven cooked celeriac chips and greens
- ❖ Coconut and lemongrass chicken escalope fried in avocado oil, green beans, cauliflower and other greens. http://cooklowfodmap.com/low-fodmap-coconut-and-lemongrass-chicken-escalopes/
- ❖ Grilled sea bream on a bed of cauliflower and onion mash, with some toasted pinenuts

Snacks

- ❖ Hard boiled eggs
- ❖ Cubes of cheese
- ❖ Double cream and berries
- ❖ Cheese crisps http://lowcarbinthe.uk/blog/cheese-crisps
- ❖ A good handful of mixed nuts, salted almonds or brazil nuts
- ❖ A couple of squares of dark chocolate.
- ❖ Salami/Pepperami
- ❖ Kabanos (Polish sausage)

- ❖ Fathead sausage roll
- ❖ Coffee with a nice splash of double cream
- ❖ Salted almonds, pork scratchings and cheese

A special note about breakfast

Through all of this, and especially after shift 7, you are probably asking "Well, what do I eat for breakfast now eh???"

Whilst I've given some suggestions already, for most people breakfast feels like pretty much the biggest challenge. For a person brand new to low carb it seems that everything that is "breakfast food" is off the menu.

In the UK, we have been trained since the 50's[21] that breakfast is usually carbohydrate based – cereal or toast/bagel/muffin/crumpet (with jam) and orange juice – as you know now, a meal that very much sets the body up to ask for more food soon after it is consumed.

However, "breakfast food" is a relatively new concept – created by marketers to sell cereals and bread in the late 19th century. Before cereal, people simply ate the food they had to hand to break their fast, with only the upper classes having more specific food offerings in the mornings, dictated by fashion rather than anything else.

All that aside, changing what you eat for breakfast may well be the most radical part of this whole transformation, so, let's take a moment to focus on what breakfast now means, with a touch of science to explain why:

---

[21] http://www.bbc.co.uk/news/magazine-20243692

Overnight, as our stomachs empty, our bodies very happily burn away our stored fats to keep us alive overnight as we sleep. If we had not evolved to do this very early on, we would have to stay awake and eat constantly. Surprisingly, we burn large amounts of energy whilst sleeping, as our bodies and our brains do a great deal of repair to themselves overnight that cannot happen whilst we are awake.

This is all powered in the main by our fat reserves. If we don't get enough sleep, our metabolism burns fewer calories overall, so that it preserves its ability to use fat to power our healing overnight.[22]

As the body mechanisms of having low carb life had us running off our body fat reserves and consumed fats rather than carbohydrates, the first meal of the day ideally contains food that enables the body to continue what it was doing overnight effortlessly.

I'll dig deep into the hormone pairs Insulin and Glucagon, Leptin and Ghrelin in part three. For now, take my word for it that this means that a meal consisting of food that

- ❖ Stimulates the satisfaction hormone Leptin
- ❖ Suppresses the hunger hormone Ghrelin
    - ○ (NB: Less sleep activates Ghrelin, as the body asks for food as energy to compensate for the lack of sleep)
- ❖ Stimulates the fat burning hormone Glucagon

---

[22] https://www.psychologytoday.com/blog/the-source-healing/201010/sleep-more-burn-more-fat

- ❖ Suppresses or does not stimulate the fat storing hormone Insulin

What effect on hormones do the macronutrients have?

- ❖ Ghrelin secretion is supressed by eating protein
- ❖ Glucagon secretion is also stimulated by eating protein, which in turn suppresses Insulin
- ❖ Low Insulin levels allow Leptin to tell the brain that no more food is required
- ❖ Fat has a mild stimulating effect on Leptin secretion, but has no effect on the secretion of Insulin
    - ○ Fat also stimulates a healthy bowel movement as well as reassuring the body that there is plentiful energy from food in the now, which means that the body is safe to continue to use up stored body fats

So, if you glossed over that part, what does this mean in practice? Eating a satisfying meal of fatty protein to start the day is awesome for you and your life. Also, sleeping well both burns body fat away and helps to keep appetite in check.

Insulin secretion is stimulated by eating carbohydrate, which, as you can see from the above, is why it's the worst thing to choose for breakfast.

So, what are the breakfast options then?

The 1950's marketing slogan "Go to work on an egg" is perfect advice. As human food, the egg is virtually perfect, containing the complete spectrum of amino acids, the right amount and quality of fats (and lecithin to aid in emulsifying it) and every mineral and vitamin you are going to need to live thrive and survive, bar Vitamin C. Eggs are a perfectly proportioned, perfect delivery system for nutrition that our bodies love.

There are only so many eggs that a person can eat though, from a mental perspective more than a physical one. Eggs, the traditional breakfast protein can get a little dull day in and day out, and this is where "thinking outside the cereal box" comes into play.

To your body, breakfast is just another meal. Your body doesn't have any concept of "breakfast food" at all and what we eat at breakfast time is linked to cultural norms, not to body requirement. To the body, all food is either energy or building blocks.

Note that you also don't have to eat breakfast if you are not hungry, despite what common wisdom says about it being the most important meal of the day. The overnight actions of ketosis I describe above can happily keep you running until much later in the day than "breakfast time" – which, if you choose to throw some intermittent fasting (IF) into your life, breakfast is usually the meal that is easiest to skip. (I'll talk about IF and why it's excellent for healing the body in the science section)

So, at the weekend, I usually skip breakfast altogether and the first meal I eat will be "lunch" or I if I am hungry, I'll have fried eggs and sausages or burgers with maybe some sort of spinach, tomato, shallot and mushroom sauté (whatever vegetables I have in the fridge), a cheese and vegetable omelette or left-overs from the night before and then only have a light snack mid-afternoon and then not eat again until evening, if at all.

As you can see, most of these foods are not at all "breakfast" but they all fulfil the criteria of satisfying hunger and encouraging Glucagon secretion. There are infinite possibilities once you crack the "breakfast is just another meal" habit.

What happens when you "fail" and why failure is a good thing.

Note I used the word when and not if and put fail in quotes - because with these steps, there is no failure, simply making choices and living life. The only failure comes from making ill-advised food choices and not learning what triggered you making that choice.

All of us make ill-advised choices from time to time, it's simply part of life. As such you will notice that I use the word avoid and not remove (except in a couple of cases, such as for alcohol, margarine and other trans-fats) as we are aiming for progress, not perfection.

Eating this way for life is about making choices, honouring self and mostly eating food that is not destructive to the body.

Making the best choices possible is simple common sense, as a non-optimal choice is immediately noticeable in terms of how it will make you feel.

There will always be times that we make a choice that is not to our body's benefit - a non-optimal food crosses our path, (and I'll freely state that mine is chips) and we have to make the choice to either eat it or not in that moment.

We all chose to make a non-optimal choice from time to time. Sometimes this choice is conscious, other times, especially of we've allowed ourselves to get too hungry, it's driven by our instincts, habit and even by our gut microbiome, and we don't realise we've made a non-optimal choice until we've nearly finished the plate!

In my case, that's ordering a side of chips in a restaurant rather than a side of vegetable or salad.

If this does happen, then deal with that choice you make as an adult. The current mentality around dieting has strong interests in keeping us in a childish mindset when it comes to food, making us a victim of our own weak will rather than to a diet that works against how we evolved.

Start now to move away from that mentality; you haven't been bad, you have done nothing wrong, you simply made a choice. Eat with no guilt, take a drink of water and simply move on to your next optimal mouthful

A non-optimal food choice is never an excuse to wreck your life. Commit to the decision to make more optimal choices than non-optimal ones, and your mind and body will work very happily together.

A blip is just that, a blip - use the skill of detached observation, which we will talk more about in part two, to learn from the experience and then move on with life.

There is also research showing that an occasional wobble is a good thing - the body is evolved to deal with "the unusual" (this activates a mechanism called hormesis) and by occasional throwing something bizarre into the mix, it helps your body to hone its response and stay optimal - it also helps you to understand the signals your body used to tell you "I didn't like that!" or "More of that stuff please!"

So, now we have sorted out the relatively easy part of what to eat, it's time to turn our attention to the more important part of this change, the keys that will unlock our minds to make the change stick.

We'll shine a light on all the past assumptions that we have picked up and how we think about food and ourselves, and then work to change our assumptions for the better.

I know this sounds scary, however, as I said earlier, if we simply change our food without also challenging and changing our assumptions and past patterns, we will simply revert to how we used to be. And that usually means ending up fat, tired and sick again.

Part two

Delving deep into our minds; why they are stacked against us, and identifying the keys and secrets to unlocking our success

"What we dwell on is who we become..."
- Oprah Winfrey

As I talked about in the introduction, the journey towards an optimal body isn't only about the food we choose to eat, it's also about the attitudes and assumptions that we consume from society as well.

This is where the challenge really starts. Until we begin to dig into how we currently think and start to actively choose a slightly different path, we are asleep to the fact that we live our lives as the sum of our past experiences - making the "same" choices over and over, simply because of the set of assumptions we have made about the world and the way that it is.

I feel that this part of the work is of greater importance than changing the food that makes our body healthier.

Without a shift away from self-hate and judgement based on impossible and two-faced standards, there is a very large chance that any change in body composition towards the healthy will simply change back again "once the diet is done".

It is also very much not "the work of a moment" – we learned the assumptions leading to our current sets of thoughts, feelings and reactions over the whole of our lives. Something that we saw, heard, felt or experienced when we were four can resonate through life without us consciously realising it. So, as you can imagine removing these assumptions takes a bit of work!

So, to start of this section, I'm going to start gently, and introduce to you the concept of resistance, and how it gets in the way of what we want.

Key 1: Resistance vs. what we want

What is resistance? It comes from our ego and is the protective force inside all of us that wants to maintain the status quo, so that we stay safe as we are and don't change and grow. Change is an unknown, and as far as the ego is concerned, the unknown is harmful to us.

The ego has an ever hungry "need to know", which can be massively useful if we have discoveries to make, but not so useful when we need to take a leap of faith and try something new because the current situation really isn't working anymore.

When an opportunity presents itself, the voice of resistance is the one that says to us "Best not do that then, just stay here in our nice little world and be secure in what we know right now" - even when we rationally want, even need, to make that change for our long-term good.

The need to "stay safe" comes direct from the amygdala, AKA the "reptile brain" which is deep inside our brain's structure. Evolutionary studies show that this part of the brain's limbic system evolved before all the other layers of the cortex. One of its jobs is to oversee our instinctual decision making and emotional response - "fight, flight or freeze" – so that we stay alive.

The amygdala bases its decision of what reaction to give to any given situation on our past experiences. Our past experiences built our ego from the age of nought to four years old. As such, the ego is a fixed structure, we cannot change it. Very useful for survival when we were children, not so handy now we are adults, and able to move on and make rational and empowering choices.

So, why is it important for us to learn to discern when this little nugget of our brain activates? Because resistance has no language or sense of time. It acts in the now to keep us alive and safe in a way that is based on our past experiences. It moves us away from pain and towards pleasure and it always points towards short term safety and satisfaction over long term gain.

As an aside, it's also responsible for weird and irrational snap decisions around instant gratification – that sweet sticky doughnut you ate even though you weren't hungry, or those lovely new shoes that you have no idea why you bought.

Advertisers and marketers play heavily to this instinctual behaviour as they create adverts and lay out shops, their jobs depend on knowing how to play our resistance to give us a short-term "happy" which increases company profits!

When we know what we want, and that progress towards a long-term change towards greater good will improve us and our world, our resistance automatically puts up "stay safe, be happy in your now, don't change" signals.

Resistance takes many shapes: fear, self-doubt, procrastination, distraction, addiction, timidity, narcissism, self-loathing and perfectionism, to name a few. I'm sure that you've feel these come up in your lives, I know I have in mine!

Procrastination is the main way my resistance shows itself, which is one reason why I didn't start on this book until late 2017, rather than in 2015 as I'd planned to do.

I have "There is a right way" and "I'm not worthy" as two of my core ego beliefs. I didn't feel that my words were worthy enough and that even if I did write them, then they had to be perfect before I could ever share them. I now know that it's better to get the words out there than to have them 100% perfect, that's what "new and revised!" editions are for!

Knowledge is power however, because we can actively gauge and use the strength of the resistance we feel against "the good thing that we want to do" - we can use it as a compass.

As Steve Pressman says in his book "Do the Work"- *'Resistance wants us to not move away from our current state of mind; it's a negative, repelling force. It will outright lie to us, fabricate reason after reason for us not to act, and cajole, seduce or bully us into not moving forward. However, Resistance, being negative, is always lying, and it is totally full of bullshit."* [23]

The fact that resistance is **always** a liar means that when we are feeling the most resistance to a new idea or

---

[23] Do the Work: http://amzn.to/2zC7jZ4

change, that is when we most need to act! Use the feelings of resistance to guide us towards the calling or purpose that we know that we must follow.

However much we want to achieve our goals towards "greater good" and "a better world", the more important that work is to us, the more we feel the resistance trying to put us off our pursuing it.

So, let's get to know what your resistance looks like about your gaining your optimal body. Take out your journal and answer these questions. (I've also put this in the "Printables" supplement.)

Don't take too long over the exercise, simply write a sentence or three on what you think and feel, and don't self-censor. You will be surprised at what's going on at the subconscious level that you don't know until you shine a light on it.

- ❖ What reservations do I have about obtaining my optimal body?
- ❖ What judgements have I made so far about anything, anyone (including myself), the choices I must make and the processes I must do to get where I'm going?
- ❖ What inner conflict have I been experiencing?
- ❖ As a result of all the above, what have I been doing so far?
- ❖ What message is this all sending to my subconscious?

Once you have done that. Let's look at what you want –
to gain your optimal body and all that entails for you.

Answer this set of questions:

- ❖ What vision do I have for my optimal body?
- ❖ What positive results do I expect from doing the
  work?
- ❖ What level of energy am I committed to
  contributing towards obtaining my results?
- ❖ As a result of all the above, what actions am I
  going to take?
- ❖ What message is this all sending to my
  subconscious?

Finally, decide where the power is. In the first set, which
is your resistance, or the second, which is what you want.
Because we all have both sets running all the time.

Our resistance shouts at us, through our thoughts and
feelings about "all of the things in the way", where what
we want, which comes from our intuition is a whisper.

All change is rooted in learning to listen to this whisper.

By drawing attention to our resistance, we begin to
neutralise its hold over us, and by then asking ourselves
what we what and what we are going to do about that, we
provide ourselves a massive power boost towards that
goal.

And yes, you can apply this approach to anything, not just to dropping your excess body fat and obtaining an optimal body.

You can use the same set of questions if you find you are having resistance over:

❖ Writing a book,
❖ lifting weights to gain muscle,
❖ learning how something works so that you are more able to support yourself in using it,
❖ designing and launching a website to share your ideas,
❖ painting, creating or drawing something and then showing it to people or
❖ embarking on a 6-month around the world adventure.

All of these things have in common a long-term change for the better. They all require short-term pain of some form that resistance wants to move us away from: planning, organising, potential financial shortfalls or simply the courage of our convictions to press on.

Now you know about resistance, you can make the choice to move on from it and, in the words of Dan Meredith, *'Get shit done."*

You won't make that choice all the time, and that's OK - we are human, and imperfect, but the fact that you can now ask yourself this simple question:

> **"Well, I am feeling all of this, and my thoughts are saying all that – but what do I want?"**

gives you a power beyond most people to accomplish gaining an optimal body and life and more importantly, to keep it.

Key 2: Start to free your "self" from your "mind"

Any person will tell you that for a change to be permanent, results remain because the behaviours to support change are constantly maintained. However, when standard dieting advice is based around food that causes hunger whilst also working against body systems, there is an extremely large chance that you are one of the people that has not been able to sustain that change over time.

And, as I mentioned in the introduction, if you are unable to comply with constant hunger, irritability and the other effects of a high carbohydrate starvation diet, the blame for the diet's failure to change the body is put firmly on the shoulders of the victim of the diet, not on the system itself.

Which, in the last 60 years especially, has led to Western society being packed full to the gunwales with judgement and self-hate. The ideals thrown at us by magazines and advertising are totally unobtainable (See the YouTube video - "Even Sally Gifford is not as beautiful as Sally Gifford" https://youtu.be/xKQdwjGiF-s) and the feelings of inadequacy caused by these ideals are backed up by deeply seated long terms society messaging around the abhorrence of being fat.

As a society, we expend massive amounts of energy hating; hating ourselves, the world, our situation, other people, you name it, we've been taught to hate on it -

mostly because we have been told that being anything other than our society's overall idealised perfection is "wrong".

And yes, every society has an ideal that differs from most other societies, as can been seen by the "Perceptions of Perfection across borders" project, run by Superdrug in August 2015, where 25 female designers were given a full body picture and asked to make it "in their opinion, more attractive to other citizens of their country." as well as the Before and After project in June 2014 by Esther Honig, where the artist gave a bare head-and-shoulders shot of herself to over 40 Fiverr photoshop aficionados in over 25 countries with the request "make me beautiful".[24]

Advertising especially gives us limiting messages everyday – stereotypes around "beauty", "age and aging", "fat people are not desirable/a joke"– the list goes on – and they are all based on the fact that advertising agencies know these stereotypes create sales.

Cash comes from sad and insecure people that want to spend money to change themselves, not people that are happy, secure and content with life!

Simply put, the messages that advertising and society gives us are not at all kind. They are designed to keep us trapped in a mode of "needing to be fixed" - they are also

---

[24]https://www.buzzfeed.com/ashleyperez/global-beauty-standards
and https://onlinedoctor.superdrug.com/perceptions-of-perfection/

not true, and as we internalise them, they keep us trapped in a negative mindset, far less able to make any sort of change, let alone change for the better.

Because whilst carrying more fat than is optimal for our skeletons and organs is not great for our health, and yes, we are starting to work on that to create a healthier body, it doesn't mean anything other than right now we are carrying around more fat than is healthy.

It's not bad, or wrong, sinful or a sign of weakness - it simply is.

The messages that we have internalised about "our weight" and "the need to be skinny" (at almost any cost) and also for women the " real women are weak and not muscled" message vs the "you cannot be a true man without muscles" message for men disempowers us and keeps us "needing a solution" that cannot be provided in the current paradigm without much pain and deprivation.

So, this key works by starting small, to create a solid foundation of observation and critical thinking[25], something that is no longer taught in state schools, as critical thinking doesn't teach a child to pass exams!

I'm using critical here in the sense of being able to objectively analyse and make discernments about a thought, feeling or concept, not in the pejorative or negative sense of criticism.

---

[25] https://en.wikipedia.org/wiki/Critical_thinking

Build your powers of critical thinking by becoming a "detached observer" of your own thoughts. Appreciate that "you" are not the anger, the hate or any of the other things that you call yourself in your mind or the labels you are carrying that were gifted to you by another person or society message.

Thoughts and emotions originate in your mind from your ego, and they can build into a rapid tumble of assumptions in an instant, but they are not your identity. They are not "you".

I'll say that again, because it's such a tricky concept to get your head around – your thoughts and feelings are not "you".

So, as a detached observer, when you catch yourself thinking something negative about yourself, click your fingers or flick your wrist and notice the thought with curiosity, rather than anger, hate or revulsion, and then allow it to pass - simply move away from it.

The thought is not you, you are having the thought; in having observed the thought, you can then choose not to wear that label.

Also, when you observe yourself feeling joy, love, or excitement, click your fingers or flick your wrist and allow yourself to be fully present in the emotion, enjoy it for what it is and then allow it to pass naturally, as all emotions do.

Our ability to observe our own thoughts and feelings is called "metacognition" and some philosophers, such as Aristotle, took the concept of metacognition as proof of our having a "rational soul" – which he defined as the lifeforce that is the essence of self with the ability to reflect and have knowledge of self, that lives within us driving our mind and body.[26]

To put it simply, we can think about thinking, but most of us don't step out of the rush of our thoughts and feelings that swamp our minds every second, and so are simply carried along with them, believing this to be what is supposed to happen, and that we are our thoughts.

By developing the skill of detached observation, we release our self from our mind, and gain the ability to add critical choice into how we behave.

Having choice is a theme that we will come back to again and again, because it's essential for our success.

And developing this skill is very much not the work of a moment, studies show that we start to have internalised thoughts at age 6 (when the adult people in our lives start to tell us that we can't just say whatever we feel like saying), and so we become addicted to living in our heads and our thoughts and feelings from a young age.

---

[26] rather than the Abrahamic religious concept of soul, as a something that is God-given, fashioned in the image of God and that can exist apart and separate to humanity beyond the physical.

So, when we first find the metacognition concepts, we have no previous skills in observing our minds and what it's doing at all.

Detached observation is a practice to be practised! Remembering to be the detached observer all of the time, or even most of the time, will in itself take time to become habit.

You will forget to do it almost all of the time to start with, but as you practise more and more, it will become second nature.

And slowly but surely, how you react to the world and what it throws at you will change, and not just in terms of how you react when people offer you a biscuit.

It's a fun ride for sure!

Key 3: Start to declutter society messaging around sugar and fat

When we start to avoid something that society has taught us is one of the keys to our happiness, how we express love, and is practically the only source of energy we need, these feelings are natural. Society gives us messaging around sugar that is neither true nor useful for our ongoing health, and our brains turn these into scripts that we use over and over again.

For instance, right about now, you may be resenting having to "give up sugary treats". This is simply because the messaging around sugar is "Sugar is love".

By avoiding sugar, your poor ol' subconscious may well be throwing up "weird to you" feelings because it thinks that it might be missing out on love because you are now avoiding one of its representations.

Think about it, the standard gift from a lover is flowers and chocolate, and we give lollipops to children when they have been good, because we love them and want to treat them. "Give me some sugar!" being the prime example of "Sugar" being a proxy for "Love" in speech, and I know I still catch myself saying "Sweet!" when I'm happy and agreeing with someone that something we have achieved is excellent (It's a particularly South London thing...)

However, the "sugar is love" message is simply not true, it's a societal fabrication with its roots coming from when sugar was an expensive resource – our bodies evolved when sweet things to eat that we can easily obtain were scarce.

It's been proved over and over that over consumption of refined sugar and carbohydrate causes us to gain body fat, mostly in studies trying to prove that either fat was the bad actor, or that the absence of fibre was the thing doing the harm.

Sugar also reduces our ability to fight off infection[27] as well as messes with a whole bunch of our hormone and lipid regulation systems.

I can't think of one set of parents I know that would willingly give their children something that is a known toxin, and yet they happily give their kids sweets, crisps, jam sandwiches, and fruit juice believing that these things are 100% safe and even healthy in some cases for their children to eat.

Conversely, fat, especially saturated animal fat and cholesterol, is sold to us as something to be avoided at all costs, a menace, a toxic substance that clogs arteries and causes our spare tyre to inflate, which in itself is a separate and pernicious primary sin to society.

---

[27] Consuming sugar lowers our Leucocytic index to nearly zero, from an average of around 13. This index is the measure of how well our immune system is working - http://askwaltstollmd.com/articles/sugarimm.php and http://www.second-opinions.co.uk/leukocytic_index.html

Yes, you guessed it, this message is also not true - there is no evidence at all that saturated fat is harmful to our body, or that it causes heart disease.

Study after study performed to try and verify the lipid hypothesis first thought of in the 1950's has failed to find any supporting evidence to validate the hypothesis, and if the results are not viewed with unfortunately human and prejudiced eyes, plenty of evidence to damn it.

As to cholesterol, it is an essential requirement in our diet, as it is incorporated into every cell in our body. Our glands make our hormones from it, brain neurons are made from it and the myelin around our nerves is 20% cholesterol[28]. If we eat less of it, our bodies simply make more to compensate for the loss of it from our diet.

Finally, dietary fat eaten in the absence of carbohydrate that is excess to body repair requirements cannot be metabolised into body fat, it is instead used as a fuel source.

So, as you can see, the messages given to us by society in the last 60 years or so are not true, and very much not at all useful.

So, start using your newly formed detached observer skills and work to notice these messages as you think them. This will give you an insight into what you then need to declutter, which as well as it being a major principle of Feng Shui, is pretty much the first step in all

---

[28] https://en.wikipedia.org/wiki/Myelin

mindset work, as having clutter hanging about confuses intent.

The clutter I am talking about here is all the assumptions we have made around sugar and fat given the information we have received on them. And yes, decluttering our physical space is also really a good thing as well, so I will be asking you to do some work on that too, but not yet.

Recognising and then working to declutter the limiting assumptions that we've unknowingly built into our world view is important; simply put, they hold us back. As Henry Ford said, *'Whether you think you can, or you think you can't--you're right."*

However much we attempt to change our diets by willpower alone, if our underlying assumptions are made out of statements that look like "sugar is love" and "all this fat will kill me!" then these assumptions will give us what's called cognitive dissonance and so make us feel uneasy about the change.

This allows resistance to kick in and so we are far more likely to eat our favourite sugary treat, even as we rationally beat up on ourselves for "yet another failure" - because we don't even know we have an underlying assumption that will win out over willpower on its own every time!

In essence: start to observe your inner thoughts (self-talk) around sugar and fat and the feelings that they generate. Also observe your thoughts and feelings about other activities that you find pleasurable that are not food based. Note these thoughts and feelings down in your journal, and get curious about them.

Ultimately, we are aiming to change our assumptions, thoughts and feelings as to what constitutes a "treat" in a world where we know that sugar is toxic! But for now, start small, hang with the tension and gain the self-knowledge - use it to fuel the work as you progress.

Also worth noting here, but I'll come back to later on in Key 7: as we grow up, our brain builds patterns to form our minds, and groups of assumptions and habits get together and form what some psychologists call "parts".

So, right now, there is the part of you that learned early on that sugar is a good energy source, and over time it's learned how to acquire the best sources for you in the easiest way possible and that fast-acting carbohydrate is very enjoyable and also gives us a short term burst release of very pleasurable dopamine.

This part of you may well be kicking up a large amount of fuss about having nothing to do right now. It's been so used to finding and acquiring fast acting sources of carbohydrates for you that us making it redundant is going to be making it rather grumpy. It will kick up a fuss and rebel against redundancy as it tries to do its job again for you.

Trying to use willpower alone isn't ever the right tactic, and I'll talk about why in a moment. For now, bear with me a little longer - observe it making a fuss and tell it out loud or in your journal what a fantastic job it does for you, how proud you are of its abilities and tenacity in seeking out sugar and carbs.

Tell it that you think it's awesome. Give it a name if you feel moved to do so, that will cheer it up no end, and when in a little while we give it another job to do, something else to be fantastic at, it will love you and will willingly undertake that new job for you with enthusiasm, now that we have shown it some love.

Talking of love...

Key 4: Practise some radical self-love: celebrate yourself and your body, as it is right now

Another thing that our western society does is hyper-sexualise the human form. For instance, consider the sharp contrast seen between people being disgusted by breast feeding in public, telling the mother to cover up and that they should be ashamed to have a breast out of clothing to feed their child, and yet not also being at all outraged that bikini clad or bare breasts or a plunging décolletage are in our newspapers and magazines, used to sell almost everything, transformed away from their actual reason for existence into marketing tools and playthings.

We are taught that our bodies in general and nudity especially is a bad thing, and that it must never be shared outside of a sexual relationship. In the extreme, we are taught that we should be ashamed of our body and its base requirements, and that divorcing ourselves from what it is telling us to do will make us better people.

This broken relationship between body and mind is a big driver to our making very non-optimal choices over how we treat it and what we feed it. Essentially, we as a society have forgotten how to communicate with a large part of ourselves.

After all, the body and the mind don't talk the same language at all, so we can't simply think our way into reconnection. Thinking and language is 100% the way of the mind.

The body's language is based in feelings and sensations. Pain, pleasure, alertness, sleepiness, hunger, satisfaction to name but a few with the language of the mind. All the things that we are told to ignore when we attempt a diet via the standard methods.

To start to reconnect your mind to your body, I would like you to take a "love bath". You are going to feel silly, and if your lessons around the body being a shameful thing were strong, your resistance is going to kick in hard, and you might well want to skip this.

Heck, you even might not be ready to do it. And that's OK, you are where you are, which is actually one of the points of this exercise - if you are not really yet ready, feel free to move on.

Park in your mind for now that reconnecting mind and body is a very valuable practice and that coming back to it when you are ready will be very rewarding in the longer term. When you are ready, this key will still be here for you.

So, with a build up like that, you might be wondering what the frilly heck a "love bath" actually is? What weird and wonderful thing am I doing to ask you to do with yourself?

A love bath is a simple celebration. It's a playful opportunity for mind and body to come together and celebrate. Another thing that we are taught to shed to "be an adult" is our acting spontaneously on our feelings. Doing silly dances and moving our body, throwing cartwheels and roly-polies or singing simply because it feels good are all acts of playful happiness and celebration of the smallest things. And we are taught to ditch them when we are told "oh do grow up!"

Both our minds and our bodies love play as a means of communication, and as adults we don't play nearly enough. So, take this opportunity and have some fun all by yourself.

Prepare a bath as you usually do. Add bubbles, bath salts or a bath bomb. Or nothing at all. If you don't have a bath, turn the shower on to the right temperature.

Next, get naked and ease into the bath or shower. Settle and relax into it for a few moments, turn off that mind of ours just for a moment, and feel the heat, the water and the simple pleasure of being in hot water.

Then, when you are ready, hold up your writing hand and praise it; touch it with our other hand and say words to the effect of: "Hand, I just want to take a moment and say thank you. I appreciate you and I love you. You've written down all these great words, picked up so many things for me and dropped the things I didn't want. I'm grateful that I have you, thank you for being my hand"

Say it out loud, so your writing hand can revel in the fact that it's being singled out for praise and thanks in front of your whole body.

Take a breath, observe how you feel and then when you are ready, move on to the next body part, in whatever order you feel fits - praise your knees, your fingernails, your feet, your breasts. Tell your hair how much you appreciate its curliness, your earlobes how cute they are and your tongue on how well it talks. Omit nothing. Praise everything. And check in with yourself on your feelings as you progress.

If you have previously hated on parts of your body, you will feel resistance in now praising and accepting them, however, the entire point of doing this is to celebrate, love and eventually accept your beautiful body, exactly as it is right now, not as it may one day become or what you wish it might be.

If you don't want to praise a part of you, then observe the feelings that are stopping you, allow yourself to feel them and then allow them to pass and do it anyway. If they are especially strong write about these in your journal later, get nice and curious with yourself about the shape of your resistance.

Once you've done the outside, work on your insides: Shower your heart with love, your kidneys with gratitude, your stomach with forgiveness and your intestines with thanks for digesting all the food you eat. Praise your blood for carrying oxygen, nutrients and hormones around your body and the glands for secreting the hard-working hormones that keep you alive.

Thank your nerves for keeping you moving and your heart beating and don't forget to thank your bones, joints and ligaments, even the old, creaky, stiff ones. In fact, especially the creaky ones, they are put through so much stuff every day and they still keep doing it day after day to the best of their ability.

Take your time with this process. We spend so little time in the space of non-sexual nudity that it may well feel very strange to linger over your body and connect with it intimately at the non-sexual level.

For some of us, this type of connecting with our body means acknowledging a bunch of self-judgements and negative inner-dialogue about what other people must be thinking about our bodies that we may well be not ready to face. If you can't go there today, again, that's ok. Do what you can do now, journal about your resistance, and work your way through it so that ultimately, you own and love all of yourself, just as you are.

If you can, I'd love for you to have your very first love bath today. Trust me, your body longs to hear you say nice things about it and praise for all its hard work!

You can also simply offer praise to yourself at any time. I often talk to my tummy; I rub it, tell it that I love it and that whilst it is doing a stellar job of carry around energy reserves, it's OK for it to be smaller now, and that I will love it just as much then as I do right now. I thank my back as I walk along the road to work for being strong that day, so that I can go into the office, and when it's hurting, I tell it that I love it anyway and that I'll rest so it can regain strength.

And yes, having love baths and praising your body is to be done at regular intervals. After all, even though you've had your body a while, every relationship needs to be worked on.

This change in your relationship with your body is new for both of you, and it needs a healthy amount of regular upkeep, just like any other relationship that we have in life.

Key 5: Willpower – never there when you need it…

I could have called this fifth key "Willpower is a lie", or even "Willpower? Might as well call it 'won'tpower'!" because it's a terribly unreliable force.

Yes, doing things by sheer force of will gets stuff done, but what no one is taught about willpower is that it's a finite resource, and so has to be managed.

The more we use it over a short time period without allowing it time to renew, the less we have available to use.

Which, as I mentioned earlier, is why relying on willpower over hunger when using a conventional diet is a recipe for disaster.

If you are continually relying on willpower to stop you eating food, your willpower reserves drain, leaving you open to eating "something naughty", which then causes judgement and hate on yourself. You swear to everyone that might listen to you that you will be good again tomorrow… and so the cycle starts all over again.

Willpower is not only used up by having to resist things, but also by simply using our minds to do even quite simple tasks.

There was a Marketing study performed at Stamford University in 1999 by Baba Shiv[29]. He divided 165 Undergrads into two groups, he asked half to memorise a two digit number and gave the other half seven digits to remember. He then sent them to another room, to tell a colleague the memorised number after which they could leave.

Between the two rooms was a corridor, where the students were offered a slice of cake ("unhealthy" / emotional choice) or a bowl of fruit salad ("healthy" / rational choice) to take with them as thanks for participating.

Of the students that had the longer number to memorise, over 63 percent of them chose the cake, compared with 41 percent of those in the two digit group. Shiv remarked on this finding *"We distracted the cognitive side so that people were more likely to go with emotional impulses."*

That this tiny extra cognitive load was just enough to sway judgement away from something seen as a more prudent choice has a staggering implication to your ability to rely on willpower if you also have a job where you have to think and make choices all day.

Having to think actively saps our reserves of willpower. Yes, we can recharge it by eating well, resting and not using it repeatedly within a relatively short space of time, but I'm sure that you will agree with me that not having to

---

[29]http://money.cnn.com/magazines/business2/business 2_archive/2006/05/01/8375932/index.htm

be in a situation where we find that our willpower has deserted us when we need some in the first place is a good thing.

As I'm sure you can guess, the key here is recognising that willpower is finite. It becomes obvious that the most effective use of willpower is being strategic about it, deploying it when we need a push on something, rather than using it constantly every day in all situations.

This is one of the reasons why I very naturally evolved the OSN scale for myself; grading by nutritive value only rather than by emotions, arbitrary calorie rules or mood at the time of choosing removes the need to use willpower constantly.

Yes, there will be times when, for instance, a slice of cake comes your way, where you might have previously used the very willpower-based phrase "I can't, I'm on a diet."

And as we all know, saying "I can't" usually leads to the self-sabotage of "but I will this time" very soon afterwards.

Instead, by saying "No thank you." you are not relying on willpower, but rather asserting a boundary.

This makes a much firmer statement, both to yourself, and to other people that are still offering you cake after your first refusal!

Women especially are taught to not assert or keep boundaries.   We are generally socialised to have "flexible" attitudes and to apologise and belittle their own opinions and beliefs if they are at odds with other peoples.

"No thank you." is a complete sentence, it needs no further justification. Everyone loves boundaries, including ourselves.

If you have never asserted a boundary before, practice saying "No thank you" in front of a mirror. Say it from the heart with meaning, and with no apology tacked onto it.

Then, if you then choose to make a non-optimal choice in that moment, it wasn't because you had already "lost the battle" or "lacked willpower", it was because you actively chose to make and own the choice.

No feeling bad or guilting yourself into "being stronger next time" over it. It was just a moment in time, and you made an adult choice to eat the cake.

And because you now aren't deploying willpower all the time, when you do need it to get stuff done, it will be there for you in spades.

Key 6: Linguistics - how our use of language holds us back

"Your words shape your world" - As you can guess from the introduction, I have very strong opinions about our use of the words "weight loss" to indicate progress towards a healthier and slimmer body - I believe that these words are entirely counterproductive.

Firstly, weight is a very non-specific term, and how much we weigh on its own does not equate in any way to how healthy we are or much body fat we are carrying around.

Take for instance BMI, which is a statistic purely based on weight and height and puts most athletes in the "obese" bracket - our weight is all of our body, not just our fat. It's fat, muscles, bone, viscera, blood, hormones, lipids, glucose, glycogen, water & the content of our stomach, bowels & bladder

Our body weight varies massively on a day-to-day basis. We can weigh one thing in the morning and easily be a kilo or two heavier or lighter at bed time!

When weight is literally the worse measure we can choose to measure progress, why are we emotionally tied to the weighing scales? Because that's the way we have been doing it for the last 2500 years or so, and it's the measure that the medical and diet industries use.

We are told to value this measure beyond all others, even though it is nonsensical to do so.

To obtain an optimal body, we really don't want to think about "weight" as a non-quantified thing, far better linguistically to target what we want to reduce - fat. This is the reason why I strongly encourage you to start using the word "fat" rather than the word "weight" - get specific, it gives better results.

Secondly, the word "loss" is linguistically a terrible choice of word for success - in all spheres of life, if we lose something it holds negative connotations; a business deal, a house or a game, small things such as our keys, one of our gloves, or a £5 note, something valuable, like jewellery or our smart phone, something tragic, such as the death of a loved one, child, parent, sibling - the strength of our emotion around loss can range from mild annoyance to total devastation.

Loss also implies that we want to find what we have lost again at some point in our lives, even when we rationally know that this is impossible. Losing something is always a negative thing, and we mourn deeply the things that we have lost forever.

So, when losing can be such a traumatic experience, why do we want to lose weight? Looking at dieting through the lens of loss and deprivation, rather than as a positive change in lifestyle sets us up to fail at the outset.

People "losing weight" even call themselves "losers" with a happiness that now deeply distresses me (I know, I called myself a loser in my youth) because linguistically, I know that people "losing weight" are usually going to find it all again, and then will be unhappy when they do (which with a low calorie, low fat diet, is an endocrinological certainty).

This is the reason why I advise choosing to describe the process using words such as

- ❖ getting rid of,
- ❖ melting away
- ❖ ditching,
- ❖ shedding,
- ❖ burning,
- ❖ dropping or
- ❖ removing.

Use a word that implies permanent removal to describe what is happening.

Things that are ditched, dropped or burnt are knowingly gone forever, and the choice we make to actively remove fat is a positive one, we want what we are removing to be gone from our life for good. It's a positive choice, made with purpose.

Put these two words together, and you can see that it makes an empowering statement. Rather than losing weight, we are getting rid of fat. Rather than losing weight, we are gaining muscle and bone density. Rather than losing weight, we are rebuilding an optimal body. Rather than losing weight, we are becoming an optimal me.

Yes, it's not quite as snappy to say "I'm shedding inches" or "I'm getting rid of my fat" initially.

It doesn't trip off the tongue as naturally our habit of saying "I'm losing weight" does – however, and I trust that you agree with me, I feel that this small and simple re-framing is one of the vital pieces of maintaining a healthy body, as we are sending positive and happy vibes to the amygdala, rather than resentful, guilt-ridden and hungry ones.

Key 7: Parts theory - behaviours and habits

The brain is a meaning seeking, pattern making, prediction organ. It stores patterns in our neurons about the things that have happened and then recalls and reuses them when it feels a similar situation happens. These patterns are what forms our mind and behaviours.

There are four stages to pattern forming AKA learning:

1. Unconscious incompetence
    o We don't know that we don't have this skill, or that we need to learn it.
2. Conscious incompetence
    o We know that we don't have this skill and start to learn it.
3. Conscious competence
    o We know that we have this skill but have to think about using it.
4. Unconscious competence
    o We don't have to think about using this skill, it just seems natural and easy.

Everything we have learned to the level of unconscious competence becomes the remit of the body to look after, not the mind, and becomes a behaviour, otherwise known as a habit.

Once we learn how, we never think about how to talk, walk, drink, eat, drive, smoke, brush our teeth, breathe, play an instrument, bite our nails, chew a pen when we think or how to get dressed. The part of our brain that holds the patterns that run the body is dealing with all of these at a level unconscious to our mind.

In fact, if we try and use our mind to think about how we do anything we have become unconsciously competent at, we become worse at it as we think about it. You can see this beautifully in the sport of cup stacking - https://youtu.be/-nhRPVWM9A0

One branch of philosophy calls our behaviours and habits "Parts" - as a part of the brain is encoded with neurons and so has learned how to do one thing and do it to excellence.

Right now, you have the habit of eating sugar and carbs - there is a part of you that learned at a young age to acquire and eat sweets or maybe large servings of bread or potatoes. It's the part of you that drives you finding yourself by the fridge at 10 o'clock at night, with no idea why you are reaching in to grab a snack - and because it has unconscious competence, it does an awesome job at seeking sugar and carbs for you to eat and it's not something that you consciously think about - it simply happens, in the same way that breathing does.

However, as you are now changing what foods you are choosing to eat, you are stopping it from doing its job, so it is almost certainly kicking up a monumental fuss! Not being able to do an assigned job makes any worker unhappy!

The key to changing an unconscious pattern is to recognise it, and then re-task the collection of neurons that make up that part.

Using the same process of learning, we do this by consciously observing how the part runs, then consciously making a change and then repeating the action until the new behaviour becomes unconscious.

As you are already doing, when you feel those cravings, tell it what a good part of you it is, so eager, so keen! Tell it that it is doing a good job and you are proud of it. All workers like to hear praise from the boss. You can even give it a name, "Sugar Seeker", "Bread Finder", or whatever you feel is a good fit for it.

Next, decide what new behaviour you would like this part of you to perform - finding optimal foods, creating focus for work, going to the gym twice a week - anything that you feel is a motivating job that will improve your life and health.

Then, get out your journal and write down the thoughts that your self-talk is having, to work out the part's current pattern.

Suggested setup phrases for this are:
- ❖ "I assume that I must have sugar because xxx"
- ❖ "Potatoes make me feel xxx so I eat them because yyy "
- ❖ "When I eat cakes, I see that xxx happens, and I eat them because yyy"

As you can see, each statement asks for your reasons, which really help you dig into and unpack the structure of the part and how it does its job. Use one of the above or think of an alternative that resonates more with you.

Once you have your statement, capture your uncensored thoughts on the page, whatever falls out of your head. Knowledge is power, and by writing you discover what triggers drive the part into action.

As with all journaling exercises, get curious and really dig in to what's going on.

Then a while later, go for a walk, preferably in nature with no tech or other brain stimulation bar the trees, wind, sunlight etc. Have an out loud conversation with this part of you. If you named it previously call it by name, and address it directly, in a curious and positive frame of mind.

As you walk, pause to listen to what feelings and sensations you get as you ask questions of it, and notice what you notice. It may be hard to hear the language of the body if you are not practised at it, but our body says stuff to us all the time, if we only pause to listen to it.

A very important point to make: no passing judgement on what feelings or sensations occur or your body's behaviours, it's only doing what it learned to do for you over time.

After a while, enthusiastically ask it to take on the new job you chose for it for you, use a phrase similar to "I know you will be equally as good at XYZ as you were at finding carbs and sugar" to seal the new thought in at the conscious level.

Once the new intention is set, repeat the new behaviour so that it sinks to the unconscious level forming a new pattern of neurons, which allows the old pattern to slowly wither and eventually die away.

A study in 2009 at University College of London (UCL)[30] found that it takes on average 66 days to train a new habit or retrain an old one, which is why I asked you to make the shift to low carb last ~39 days. By taking this time, I'm getting you half way to the new habit already!

Pattern rebuilding takes doing the new behaviour more than either the old behaviour or not doing anything at all. New patterns are formed by consistent action. You don't have to be perfect, but you do have to act.

Have a conversation with your "Sugar Seeker" quite often, especially if you feel yourself wanting some sugar for no particular reason at all. Once you have re-trained this enthusiastic worker to have another role, it will be as happy and marvellous as its new job as it was about finding you sugar and carbs to eat.

Also worth noting in particular reference to physical sugar cravings, taking the supplement Chromium Picolinate at a dosage of 200 mcg a day helps to regulate

---

[30]http://www.ucl.ac.uk/news/news-articles/0908/09080401

our carbohydrate metabolism, and so removes physical sugar cravings.

Once you've done that, it then really all is about recognising and retraining new patterns.

I note here that if you replace sugar filled confection with low carb replacements, this is not retraining your old patterns and will keep your "Sugar Seeker" fully employed in their old role, which means it will be working against what you rationally want to happen.

Key 8: Change from a "stuck structure" that will never work to get results

One of the great disservices that our brains and so society gives us is the want for opposites. The world is filled with shades of grey, but our brains are wired to work in absolutes. Our philosophers have been thinking about this since around 525BC, the concept flowed over to the scientific method and so western society expects simple stark duality from the world, rather than reality, which is something far more complex to resolve[31]

However, when we work towards a change, it is this polarity that trips us up. As Albert Einstein said, '*We cannot solve our problems with the same level of thinking that created them*' and if we look at a standard reason for "weight loss" - "to be thin" - we can see that this comes from a place of "the opposite of what we don't want" - "to be fat"

"To be thin" and "to be fat" are the opposite of each other, and so both come from the same level of thinking. They cancel each other out, which unfortunately results in our staying the same as we always are.

To avoid this, a re-frame of our outcome is required, so that we "rise above" the current issue to create the best possible outcome for ourselves. The challenge is to be able to frame the outcomes so that it elevates and

---

[31] https://en.wikipedia.org/wiki/Unity_of_opposites

enlivens us, rather than leaving us mired in the problem and its mere opposite.

Therefore, I have my personal best outcome set currently as: "living an optimal life", which I trust that by the end of this book you will share with me in some way. This is an outcome in and of itself, it is not dependent on my situation, moods or anyone else and is certainly not an opposite of anything.

There is an exercise that you can do to aid you in finding out your own best outcome

Problem →
Impact of the Problem →
Desired Outcome →
Best Outcome

So that you can see how this might work for you, I've filled in a matrix as an example.

Take your journal and fill out the below for yourself
(A blank copy is in the printables supplement):

Problem	❖ I'm fat. I don't want to be fat.
Impact of the problem	❖ I cannot easily buy clothes. ❖ My hip and knee joints ache so my focus suffers at work. ❖ However much I restrict what I eat, I never seem to get any smaller. ❖ I'm constantly "on a diet" and I'm always hungry. ❖ I worry about what other people think of me ❖ I worry about what impact being fat has on my health. ❖ I'm single and I don't date, because I'm too afraid of being rejected. ❖ I feel like I get passed over for promotion at work, based on how I look.
Desired outcome / Absence of the problem	❖ I eat healthy nutrient dense food that satisfies, so that I never feel deprived ❖ I easily buy clothes that fit well and look fabulous. ❖ I have less pain ❖ I have more focus.
Best outcome	❖ I am able to open my heart and find a long-term partner that accepts me. ❖ My boss relies on me more and I get the promotion that I've been wanting for a few years. ❖ I am confident that I have a healthy body, and that I will live a long and happy life

Use present tense for all of boxes, this ensures that your mind accepts what you have written more readily. As you can see, the reframe to best outcome bears little resemblance to the initial problem.

Whilst the "opposite of what you don't want" can be a useful springboard for inspiration, it's simply a stepping stone to your best outcome.

Key 9: Moving from limiting to empowering assumptions - stories and self-talk

We are given limiting messages that become our shared values everyday - "self-control is the way to lose weight" is the one that I'll talk about here.

Just as with behaviours and habits, our beliefs (core identities), values (a shared/society belief) and assumptions (how we expect ourselves and other people to behave be based on our own beliefs) are also laid down as neuron patterns in our brain.

The brain encodes beliefs, values and assumptions from what happens around us and to us. It then uses these constructs to create stories that continually reflect and re-enforce the constructs.

"What you see is what you get" has literal meaning to the brain. As much as seeing is believing, believing is seeing.

For instance, a negative "If... then" statement about something that happened and our reaction to it could create the assumption "If I eat the cake, then they will think I have no self-control" The assumption is created and then our self-talk gives it back to us when we are offered cake.

If this behaviour repeats often, then a limiting and negatively framed identity belief gets coded - "I'm a greedy screwup"

So, when we eat cake, we feel guilt over eating the cake, as we are breaking a value that has been imposed on us by messaging - "self-control is the way to lose weight."

However, all of this negative self-talk is simply stories we tell ourselves built from what we assume to be true to allow us to conform to society norms. They are the habits of past behaviour, and they can be reprogrammed in the same way as our physical behaviour

This simple to understand, but not so easy to do though. This stuff is embedded deep in our ego, which as I said back in key 1, is a fixed structure built on the stories we made up from our experiences as a very young child.

We build stories around the most seemingly innocent of things. Something as innocuous as you overhearing a nursery assistant telling your parents "he seems to be more of a follower than a leader" or hearing a snarky family member remarking at a family gathering "she's very loud, isn't she?"

And of course, the stories we make are protective, designed to keep us safe so that we survive and as we have discussed, this protection the root of our resistance and so is often framed negatively. The name that psychologists give this voice is "the inner critic"

It's the voice that runs us down, tells us to not try, that we are not worth it, not good enough, too fat, too poor, too ugly, won't achieve anything of value, don't belong, aren't capable, don't have the capacity – you know that voice, you almost certainly listen to it constantly.

It's the voice that insults us at every opportunity, and yet, if what we say to ourselves were said to us by someone external, most of us would not stand for in any way shape or form, would confront the person telling us such nasty things and tell them in no uncertain terms of stop and/or go away!

Everyone has an inner critic, and for most people, those that haven't started to do the type of work that we are doing around the way our minds work, it runs our lives on autopilot.

I'll talk about one of my deeply embedded stories "If I'm small I will get hurt" and how that was holding me back in a very tangible manner in a little while. Because I was listening to my inner critic telling me not to do stuff and acting based on that message, all without me realising it, this book nearly didn't get written.

So, know now that the inner critic is part of your resistance. Using the same skills of detached observing, we can know with rock solid certainty that it is talking bullshit.

Get that journal out again and get intensely curious! Figure out what emotion is behind each of the stories your inner critic comes up with.

Are you scared? Angry? Sad? Then, figure out what pattern of behaviours is triggering your inner critic to activate

The inner critic will always be there, but we don't have to listen to it or act on what it is saying. Greet it, acknowledge it and let the voice yatter on until it shuts up because you aren't listening any more.

Tune it out and silence it by not getting wrapped up in the story it is telling you. Because the story is utter, total and complete bollocks. You don't have to act on what it is saying, as an adult, you have that choice.

Knowing this is only half the key though – the other half is to start to nurture our "inner advocate"

Again, we all have one, it's the voice that supports what we want. The whisper of inspiration, the support for the things that we are here to achieve.

Your inner advocate is there to encourage you with the truth which reflects the gifts you bring to this world.

Just like the inner critic is the voice of all your detractors, the inner advocate is the voice of your greatest supporters. The champions in your life and what they would say to you to about how wonderful and resilient you are.

The inner advocate has a quiet voice, which is why more often than not it gets drowned out when we are too busy in being wrapped up listening to the yell that is our inner critic.

However, the inner advocate is certain, sure and implacable once you start listening to it, and it's from this place that we work to rebuild our assumptions

Instead of deflecting complements (and women especially are socialised to do this so much, it's seen as unseemly to accept the complement) start to simply say thank you and use the comment to begin to transform the positive feedback you receive from others into the confidence to listen to your inner advocate.

Once you start to acknowledge that the light that others see you in is nowhere near as harsh as your inner critic would tell you that you are, and in fact most of the people that you know and love actually think you are pretty awesome[32], the inner critic begins to lose its power, allowing you, for maybe the first time in your life, to be supported by both your inner advocate and your friends, families and chosen families.

It's always easier to achieve anything we set our minds to with support. Going it alone is always a harder path. And when we are divided against ourselves by our inner critic, we are very much on our own.

---

[32] Notwithstanding some of the tricky and rather negative relationships that family can sadly sometimes have.

Key 10: Developing the deeper conversation between your mind and your body through love

Love your tribe

Whenever we make a dramatic change in our life, there's a natural temptation to evangelise about it and help friends and family enjoy meaningful breakthroughs of their own. However, the reality is that people will only change when they're ready.

They will in some cases literally not hear you or will totally misunderstand you if you try to tell them something they are not ready to receive. This is nothing to do with you, it's simply how the mind works.

Apparently, snakes feel the same way. For years herpetologists tried to discern when snakes will shed their skin but have never been able to discover a pattern to it.

Nothing in a snake's genetics or environment gives any clues about when or why they'll shed. So, researchers settled on the most obvious answer: Unlike dogs that shed regularly twice per year, or chickens which moult every autumn, snakes shed their skins when they want to shed them. It simply happens when the snake feels like shedding, and it isn't at all externally influenced.

So, the best way to encourage others towards change is to inspire them through our own successes and growth. As your friends start to notice your size reduction, the glow of your healthy skin and the light in your eyes, they will take you aside and ask what you are doing!

No person will change until they are ready. Until that moment arrives, until they specifically request your advice on making changes in their own life, the best way to support other members of your tribe is simply to love them.

Love them as unconditionally as you are now loving yourself… just the way they are right now. Shine light and love on them and then if they decide to let go of carbohydrates and their excess body fat in their own time, then offer your support in that goal generously and unequivocally.

Note that there will always be people in your tribe that will never reach that tipping point. And that's okay. That's their journey through life. Your only job is to love them and support them and be there for them just the way they are as they are right now.

Love your body

Most of us spend large sums of money and time on informing and/or entertaining our minds. To feed our minds we invest in all manner of books, magazines, films, television shows, the internet, Facebook, Netflix, Amazon Prime, iTunes etc., yet we very much skimp when it comes to feeding our bodies. Given how we are conditioned to view them, this is not at all surprising.

One fact that we must face when making the shift to a low carb lifestyle is that nutrient dense ingredients cost more money than non-optimal carbohydrate-based processed foods.

One of the best ways to love our body is to always buy the best quality food we can afford. Yes, this is a sliding scale for all of us, and having been in a place of "no extra cash", I lived through that experience myself – and one of my next books is going to be all I can think of on the "low carb on a budget" topic.

However, it's not that nutrient dense food "costs too much", it's that subsisting off cheap carbs costs us too little, both in terms of the money we pay for it as well as the wider health of our environment.

There is also a growing body of evidence shows that our beneficial gut bacteria support positive mood and emotional well-being and yet the steady diet of junk food that society would have us eat actively kills off our gut microbiome.

As society has changed, so our priorities have changed. In the 1980's the average UK family spent anywhere from 15 to 25% of their income on food.

By 2010 this had dropped to 10%. One of the reasons we're in the midst of our present obesity nightmare is that we've been spending too little on our food.

It does seem that as a society, although more so in America than in the UK, the less we spend on our food, the bigger our waists become. Sugar and processed carbs cost next to nothing to produce and create a huge amount of profit for food companies, even when sold cheaply.

Let's take the example of pizza. Essentially "cheese on toast with tomato sauce." Yet, the average margarita pizza costs around £12-15 in a restaurant or for delivery.

Yes, there are restaurant overheads to consider, but even a supermarket family size pizza costs around £5.00. For ingredients that cost at maximum a pound, if that.

Show some love to your stomach and your waistline and spend money on real food for your body rather than giving all your time and money to the service of your mind.

I know people that will spend £2000 on a ticket to a self-improvement course, stay in a £100 a night hotel for days on end, yet they go out of their way to subsist largely on the hotel buffet and junk food to save money (I've done this myself in fact a few years back! Not sugary junk, "low carb junk food" but it's still the same principle)

When I suggest dropping a few extra pounds on food in order to drop a few extra pounds from your body, I'm not even talking about shopping at the farmer's market or buying organic all the time.

Yes, you can do that for even better results, but for now, aim to buy and eat quality food that needs you to do little prep – vegetables, meat, fish, fowl and eggs - and feel how much you light up with all the excess energy and vitality teeming up from within! Look at your skin and see how much more resilient it becomes, and how you gain an inner glow of health.

Love your self

You are a most amazing, beautiful and unique creation! There is no one on the planet like you.

How does my saying that to you make you feel? Hopefully, by now, not as uncomfortable as if I'd said it point blank back in the introduction!

One of the most tangible ways to demonstrate our own love to ourselves is through treating our unique beautiful body with tender loving care. If you haven't already taken your first love bath, right now would be a very good time to do so.

Make plans around sending your body the message that you love it - Book in for a massage, an alternative healing session or a yoga class. Any exercise or therapy where you actively engage in sensations and feelings of bliss/euphoria/relaxation. These types of activity send a powerful message to our bodies - "I care about you!" - in a language that the body understands.

Any day is a good time to appreciate and love your body, and the more communication that you have with it, the easier it will be to "hear" what it is saying back to you.

A more intangible way to love our self is to treat our minds well; fill them with educational things, love for our family and friends, epic experiences and being kind to those around us, rather than filling up time with televisual and other media "junk food" and negativity.

Every action we take is driven by the meaning we give to our focus about what is happening. If our focus is negative, we will give something a negative meaning and then probably take no action.

For instance, if you hold a door open for someone at work, and they breeze through in their own world without acknowledging you or saying thank you, you could focus on how impolite there are, giving the event the meaning that holding the door for such a rude person was not worth it, leading to the action of you becoming more selfish, not holding doors open, or treating that work colleague in more stand-offish fashion.

Or, you could focus on the possibility that your colleague it under pressure to deliver something, or they have had some bad news. This gives the event the meaning that you helped them with a small altruistic act, making their life that little bit easier. This could lead to the action of checking in with this colleague later, showing them some human connection, making both of you more fulfilled humans.

By treating both our minds and our bodies well, our self is not caged in by either one. Which then allows us to get on with the life we are destined to have and create the things and experiences that we are destined to create in this world.

After all, there are no spare humans, and we are all here to contribute our own unique talents to this world. Once you show your self some love, that talent can shine.

Hang on, wait a minute. That's not what you said earlier…

Yes, I said earlier that it's impossible to influence the domain of the body by thinking about it, i.e. using the mind to try to control the body. So, you might think that I've contradicted myself with a few of the keys, as they can look a little like I'm asking you to attempt to do just that.

However, we aren't using thinking to influence the body, we are ensuring that both mind and body are pulling in the same direction for the good of the self. Everything works so much better when mind and body are in communication and united in purpose.

I spoke in Key 2 about freeing your "self" from your mind, and about metacognition, the ability to think about our thoughts. I also spoke about Aristotle's thoughts on the "rational soul" and I asked you to observe and write about your thoughts, as well as your feelings and also what you are noticing about what sensations and signals the body sends when it wants you to do something.

So, the Shifts and the Keys are really all about getting you to a place where you can see that you are neither your mind nor your body.

"You", your Self, contains both your mind and your body, and that there is a communication gap between them that we need to overcome to achieve long term success.

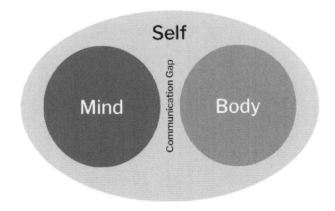

I found this out for myself at the beginning of 2017. From early 2011 to mid 2016. I was in a relationship where we loved each other with food. Consequently, I ate way too many sub and non-optimal meals for the comfort of my body.

I also had a drop in my exercise levels from a slipped disc at the end of 2012 and all this added up with me carrying around rather a large amount of excess fat again. So much in fact that I was back up to around 19st and my size 24 clothes were getting tight.

Once I broke from the relationship, I dived deeper into personal development and qualified as a coach and NLP practitioner in November 2016. Shortly after qualifying, I brought myself fully back to making optimal food choices again, even to the extent of shedding my 2.5 litre a day diet coke addiction.

I dropped back comfortably into my size 22 clothes very quickly, and then my body stubbornly sat at the same size and weight, around 18st 7lbs, until February 2017.

It was then that I did some mind work with a coach and discovered that I had what's known as an incongruency. Unknown to me, my past meant that I'd picked up the assumption that if I were to be small I would get hurt, yet I also had resistance towards appearing on video and even writing this book, because I felt I was too large to do so and have any credibility at all.

So, whilst rationally I wanted to be small, my past assumptions were blocking this. Once we brought it to light and cleaned up the assumptions I'd made, I effortlessly dropped to a size 20, without changing my food. As of July 2018, I've been hovering around the 17st mark for the last year on the scale, but my body has continued to shrink and is now comfortable in size 18 clothes.

And whilst I know that scale stalls have to happen for health, (I'll talk about this in part three) looks like I may well have some more assumption decluttering work to do on myself for the next drop to a size 16 eh?

However, getting mind and body working together can occasionally be a touch challenging, so, I'm going to let you in on three secrets that will help and guide you towards this.

Secret 1: Keep on keeping on

Even with the best will, structures and actions, you are going to revert to old patterns and behaviours initially. As I said in Key 7, it takes on average 66 days for a new pattern to embed itself and become habit.

So, what do you do if you suddenly find yourself halfway through eating something non-optimal and have no real clue why? You stop and use some detached observation to dig at what triggered the pattern.

Use your journal and ask yourself some "coaching questions" – Start with "what" or "how", as finding out what is more helpful to discovery.

- ❖ What happened there?
- ❖ What was the situation?
- ❖ Was it the food that triggered me, or something else?
- ❖ What was I feeling?
- ❖ Did anyone contribute to the trigger being activated?

Coaching questions rarely start with why – the word why can be accusatory, and so in asking "why…?", defensive and dishonest answers occur.

As I said earlier, the brain is a meaning seeking, pattern making, prediction organ. If you ask it questions, it will give you answers. Asking ourselves better questions means we get better answers!

The only failure is not learning from what happened, so that you can gradually work to change your reaction when the pattern is triggered again in the future.

Secret 2: Go clear the junk!

This secret is all about ease. Until your new patterns and behaviours are firmly embedded, there is a war going on in your mind between the old patterns, society messaging and the new ideas I've introduced to you.

So, clearing out the junk food is your insurance policy against easily falling back to an old sugar seeking pattern. Progress towards any goal becomes far easier. when you clear the house of junk. Decluttering the physical environment of the things that are not serving you is always a good thing.

When you are able to make optimal choices easily at home, you start reprogramming your mind with no effort. Which then makes the situations outside of home where you are offered a non-optimal food that much easier to deal with.

When friends and family encourage non-optimal choices, politely decline. As I said back in Key 5, "No thank you." is a complete sentence. You do not need to justify to anyone the choice you are making.

I'll note here that this secret may well be making you squirm a little. You are possibly resisting taking this action, even maybe saying to yourself that you **need** to have the junk around for your partner/guests/kids.

I'm going to challenge that assumption.

As I mentioned in Key 3, one of the main messages around sugar is that it is love. I challenge you to challenge that assumption. There are many other ways to show love and I ask you to never love anyone with sugar, including yourself.

I also said that I can't think of one set of parents I know that would willingly give their children something that is a known toxin. Sugar is a toxin, so what would motivate you feed it to your children or your partner or friends? What would drive you to ensure that their lifespan is shortened and also more likely to be filled with bad health?

And if you are a loving caring partner or parent, the answer to both of these questions will be something along the lines of "Nothing at all would motivate me to harm my partner or children! What kind of mindless freak are you to even ask me that question?!"

As you can see, you are not a bad person if you deprive your partner or your children of poison. Quite the opposite in fact.

Yes, children need nutrient dense sources of carbohydrate to fuel their growth, usually about 100 to 150g per day, as well as lovely protein and fat from which to build their body and brain. There are plenty of carbohydrates that you can give them that aren't sugar or refined flour junk. Empty processed sugar and white flour foods are simply that, empty.

Secret 3: Listen to your body – it knows what it wants

As I mentioned in Key 1, the mind lies to us constantly. However, the body never lies, it doesn't even know what the concept of lying is, as it has no words! It will feed you sensations, and at that moment in time, they are 100% true for your body.

However, a diet filled with refined carbohydrates mess with its ability to communicate clearly. Once you remove the carbs, your body's natural hormonal responses to food kick back in (I'll talk more about this in the science section), and as we learn to start listening to what it is telling us, we can be 100% sure that it is asking for exactly what it needs.

As I talked about in Key 4, we are coming from a place where we've been taught to distrust and ignore our body's signals. Learning to trust our body is a big deal.

But it's the secret to bridging the communication gap and feeding both your body and your mind with exactly what they need for you to live an optimal life.

Second guessing yourself - "Is this OK?"

Even with my giving you the OSN scale and saying that listening to your body is a good thing, if you find yourself asking this question before you make a choice, or even while you are eating something, it is probable that your past patterns have taught you to seek the validation of others above the validation of your own instinct and knowledge, essentially you've been trained by circumstance to doubt yourself.

So, if this is you, this journey will also build your own resilience. Trusting your body and listening to its feedback is potentially a new thing to you, and it's natural that building that relationship will take time.

Find the best ways to work with yourself so that you can get into the habit of believing yourself. This could be following a menu-plan to the letter (and my first book, "Control Your Low Carb Week" http://amzn.to/2hgdcBT is all about menu planning!), freestyling from a selection of food that you love and want to try out (which is my style of living a low carb life), or yes, even initially using food macros counting tools and maybe even "going keto" to give you an idea of the shape of this new way of eating to boost your confidence in making optimal choices.

And once you've found the optimal way that suits you and your life, it's then a simple matter of doing that, over and over and over. Keep on keeping on, through the blips, the trips, the stumbles and the triumphs.

And one thing that supports me in this "keep on keeping on" mode is knowing the hard science about how the body works that backs my way of life, rather than the myths, mystery and even lies that the media and government has fed us in the last 60 years.

Part three

All of the science!

'The urge to simplify a complex scientific situation so that physicians can apply it and their patients and the public embrace it has taken precedence over the scientific obligation of presenting the evidence with relentless honesty.

'The result is an enormous enterprise dedicated in theory to determining the relationship between diet, obesity, and disease, while dedicated in practice to convincing everyone involved, and the lay public, most of all, that the answers are already known and always have been—an enterprise, in other words, that purports to be a science and yet functions like a religion."

- Gary Taubes

Welcome to the section that has more information about how the body works than you ever knew you wanted to know!

As I mentioned in the introduction, I'm a logic-based individual, so I love diving deeply into all the details, unpicking how systems work and so really understanding what's going on in the body.

I fully understand if you want to skip this part totally, dip in to the things that interest you, or even skim read it for the salient details. I've connected the sections for flow as much as possible, but some of them are naturally stand-alone facts and advice that don't fit easily into a narrative.

However you approach this section, it's full of good stuff that I trust you will find useful for when you have questions and to answer other people's questions; for instance, "Why are your eating choices different to what we get told all the time?" or the heartfelt if misplaced opinion "Gosh, all that meat and fat will kill you won't it?!"

This is the section that will pull the wool away from your eyes as to why the "standard dieting advice" of the latter half of the 20th century has failed humanity over and over again for the last 60 years.

Let's dive right into the main attraction, shall we?!

It's all about hormones

Hormones are the main drivers for all body functions. Produced by the various glands in the exocrine and endocrine system, they are the chemical messengers that regulate everything that our body does. Think of the system as a symphony, all the regulatory systems working together to produce a harmonious and healthy whole. It is impossible to change one system independently of the others, if one element changes, all the others must change as well to maintain overall balance.

I'll observe here that, whilst I am a 100% fan of modern medicine and the fantastic things that it does, I feel that that our classification and separation of "each disease is an issue in itself", rather than looking holistically at the whole system and its imbalances is a major issue with our current "health system".

Most of our hormones work in pairs, one hormone that "increases" and another that "decreases", and in working to gain the body that we evolved to possess, understanding this and how these hormones interact with each other is vital.

The other thing that is vital to understanding is how we can ensure that we are promoting the production of hormones that decrease both hunger and our capacity to store fat whilst also promoting the hormones that increase energy usage via liberating fat from our fat stores.

The pair that drives blood glucose regulation and fat storage are Insulin and Glucagon, both produced by the pancreas in response to the food we eat. If I asked you what Insulin is, you would answer something along the lines of "it's that stuff that diabetics inject isn't it?" but you possibly won't know why, and you probably haven't heard of Glucagon at all.

The primary job of this hormone pair is to regulate our level of blood glucose and keep it within a very precise and narrow range.

❖ Insulin removes glucose from the blood and shoves it into muscles and fat cells when the level of "free glucose" is too high,
❖ Glucagon pulls glucose from our muscles into our blood when the level of "free glucose" is too low.

The hormone pair also control our fat storage.

❖ Insulin keeps our "not-needed for energy" triglycerides locked into our fat cells,
❖ Glucagon pulls triglycerides from our fat cells to use as energy as needed if there is little glucose in the blood to meet energy needs.

Glucagon pulling triglycerides from our fat cells is what happens overnight when we've finished digesting dinner. If we hadn't evolved storing & liberating fat for energy capabilities, we would have evolved to never sleep and would have to be constantly eating to stay alive.

When we eat starchy carbohydrate, the actions of the enzymes in our stomach break it down into glucose, which then starts to wander around our body in our blood so that Insulin can push it into our muscles, so we can then start to extract energy from it. Note that sugar, AKA sucrose, is a half glucose half fructose molecule, and fructose has a different metabolic pathway, which I'll dive into a little later.

As you can imagine, this means that we require Insulin to also run around in our blood, to precisely control how much free glucose we have running about.

Over time eating a highly processed carbohydrate-based diet there is always excess blood glucose running about. This means that Insulin "has to go in mob-handed" as it is needed in greater and greater amounts to push the same amount of excess glucose from the blood into the muscles.

This having to go in mob-handed to get the same effect is medically called "Insulin resistance" and is the precursor to type II diabetes.

In this state, the amount of glucose in our blood stays at the higher end of the required range, this also means that that we don't need much, if any, Glucagon to be active.

We are meeting glucose needs via eating almost constantly, and so we have no need release any energy from either our muscles or our fat cells.

Elevated Insulin also slows down fat burning via its indirect suppression of one of the major fat burning mitochondrial enzymes, Carnitine Palmitoyl Transferase (CPT-1)[33]

So, all this means that Glucagon becomes redundant and sits around in the pancreas twiddling its thumbs, taking it easy until way after bedtime, when Insulin can finally have a little break and Glucagon can go out to work releasing fat from our fat cells to be used as energy and stop us from dying in our sleep.

The other hormone pair to be interested in are Leptin and Ghrelin. This pair have a major influence on energy balance.

Leptin is what's called a "long-term mediator" – it tells the brain that our fat cells are full and so regulates hunger over time. It's produced mostly by our fat cells[34] to signal when they are full. It tells the brain (specifically the hypothalamus) that we have enough energy stored and that we don't need to eat anymore.

Whereas the fast-acting Ghrelin is produced in the lining of the stomach when it is empty, sending up a signal to the hypothalamus to start eating.

However, if there is lots of Insulin running about, Leptin's action on the hypothalamus is blocked, it cannot be "heard" over the amount of "noise" Insulin is making.

_____

[33]https://en.wikipedia.org/wiki/Carnitine_palmitoyltransf erase_I

[34] as well as a little in the stomach, heart, placenta, and skeletal muscle

So, there comes a point when your brain thinks it's starving even though there is ample energy hanging out in our fat cells, and so the brain drives us to eat more carbohydrate to create more glucose to satisfy its false need for energy.

As these systems get more and more out of kilter, the effects are more and more amplified, which leads to a premise that will blow your mind a tiny bit...

We don't become fat because we eat too much food.

We eat too much food because we are fat.

Being fat is not your fault, and it never was. Getting our hormones working the way that nature intended is the goal of eating a diet that is low in unnatural processed carbohydrate.

Once there is not excess glucose running about in the blood, Insulin can stop running itself ragged. Glucagon can come out to play and release energy from our fat cells and Leptin can again be heard by the brain, which gives us the added boost of lower levels of hunger.

Sounds good, doesn't it? Well, that's how our bodies are meant to work, how they evolved. With the currently recommended diet, we are "sticking our fingers in our ears and going 'la-la-la!'" and medicating our way around the issues that we've caused by moving away from what nature planned for us as we evolved.

Apart from these two hormone pairs, the other hormone that gives us pause for thought is Cortisol, the primary glucocorticosteroid secreted by your adrenal cortex. Unfortunately, Cortisol does its vital jobs at a cost to other systems that the body works to balance at all times.

It peaks in the morning shortly after waking to give us a boost to get us going (called the "dawn phenomenon[35]"), which it creates by breaking down a little protein from our muscles, liberating the building blocks for energy and body repair; glucose, fatty acids, and amino acids and making them readily available in our blood for our body to use.

Having done the job of getting us going, Cortisol levels gently drop during the day.

Because most bodily cells have Cortisol receptors, it affects many different functions in the body. Cortisol can help control blood sugar levels, regulate metabolism and it even assists with memory formulation. It also has a controlling effect on sodium and water balance and helps control blood pressure.

It's our main natural anti-inflammatory agent and maintains a balance – for any physical body to remain in homeostatic equilibrium every inflammatory reaction must have an opposite and equal anti-inflammatory reaction.

---

[35] https://en.wikipedia.org/wiki/Dawn_phenomenon

Its action keeps gnat bites from turning into huge lumps, it is the natural actor against allergens that cause bronchial tubes to swell shut, and it stops mild cat scratches from looking like you have just had a close call with a tiger.

Having it running around is essential to life, however, as with most things in life, we can have too much or too little of a good thing.

Low Cortisol causes weakness and fatigue, however high Cortisol has a much bigger impact. If we live in a state of "continual stress" - not getting enough sleep, being in a noisy environment, eating sugar and other junk that causes inflammation, being constantly "switched on" for work and paying persistent attention to social media - the persistent elevation in "baseline Cortisol" acting on the inflammatory factors coming in suppresses our immune response and wastes away our muscle tissue.

When we are under stress, our body produces Cortisol, so that we have energy available to deal with whatever is coming. Which in days gone past was a good thing, but in the 21st century, where constant stress is a factor of life, it really isn't serving us.

Another major factor in how Cortisol acts in the body is governed by which other hormones it's hanging out with as it is running around our system.

When Cortisol is hanging out with Insulin, they antagonise each other, which leads to even more fat storage.

❖ Insulin and Cortisol together increase the activity of the major fat storing enzyme, lipoprotein lipase (LPL) to a far greater extent than either does acting on its own.

❖ Insulin suppresses Cortisol's action on the major fat burning enzyme hormone sensitive lipase (HSL).

❖ This means Insulin accentuates Cortisol's LPL effect and dampens its HSL effect increasing the storage of fat while at the same time decreasing its release.

❖ Elevated Cortisol also makes the body more Insulin resistant. This means the body will need to release even more Insulin to get the job done.

However, when Insulin levels are lower, and Cortisol hangs out with Human Growth hormone (HGH), the catecholamines (Adrenaline and Noradrenaline) combination both speeds fat release and elevates fat burning.

❖ This state occurs during intermittent fasting and during short duration high intensity exercise. This is why short, overnight fasts or day fasts (i.e. 12-24hours), and short duration very high intensity workouts (i.e. 20 minutes of sprint training) can be are very beneficial. (I'll talk about intermittent fasting and exercise in more detail later)

❖ High intensity exercise stimulates a burst release of Cortisol, which is protective to our systems. Lowering Cortisol during high intensity exercise is a really bad idea but encouraging it to naturally fall away at a good pace post exercise by leading a less stress filled life can aid the anabolic/catabolic balance in the body.

❖ Eating and doing a relaxing activity following intense movement helps to ensure Cortisol levels fall quickly after intense exercise. The use of performance supplements such as Branched-Chain Amino Acid (BCAA) or whey protein also encourage this behaviour in the body.

Finally, we must think about our sex hormones. The balance of androgens and oestrogens dictate where the body fat is going to end up on our bodies. And yes, everyone has both sets of hormones in differing amounts – it's how much of each we have that determines our gender, perhaps even more than what sex organs we have. (A debate for another book entirely!)

Biologically female bodies tend to stash fat primarily subcutaneously, in the breasts, thighs and buttocks, with the stomach and visceral area around the organs as a secondary repository whereas biologically male bodies have minimal subcutaneous storage, and tend to pack their fat primarily into the visceral area, where it unfortunately squashes organs and raises the risk of heart issues.

Female bodies are also more naturally lipophilic as we evolved with the tendency for ample subcutaneous fat storage for ease of being able to produce milk for raising babies.

The change in sex hormones as we age is a massive factor which dictates a shift in fat storage locations.

In male bodies, the drop in Testosterone levels that happens with age decreases muscle mass and encourages the pot-belly effect of a solid core of visceral fat covered in an added layer of subcutaneous fat.

This happens because subcutaneous fat storage is encouraged by Oestrogen, which both sexes have but in male bodies is present in tiny amounts. The Testosterone drop amplifies Oestrogen's effect on the male stomach area, and as subcutaneous fat storage increases, so does the production of Oestrogen.

Perimenopausal female bodies shift their preferred fat storage location to the stomach and visceral areas. The body also actively starts to gain subcutaneous fat to protect its own interests; as the ovaries start to slow down the flow of Oestrogen, the female body turns to its fat cells to prop up flagging Oestrogen levels.

All these hormonal factors affect how our bodies store fat, which is one reason why two people can eat the same food yet have drastically differing results in terms of body composition.

The food we eat has an immediate and drastic effect on our hormones, and the standard diet of the last 60 years has been actively putting our hormonal systems very much out of whack.

A low carbohydrate way of life restores our balance to the state that evolution intended over time. In some people it's very much not a quick fix, but then, healing isn't instantaneous in any body.

Why a calorie is not a calorie to the body

One of the major reasons a low carb way of eating is seen as controversial is that you can do it with no calorie counting at all. Instead, trusting and listening to your body signals and eating to the point of no hunger but no further. You may have noticed that I haven't mentioned calories very much at all until this section.

The calorie was invented at some point in the 19th century as a unit of heat energy (it's invention is attributed to various people), and the "kilogram calorie" AKA Calorie with a capital C was applied to food in the US in the late 19th century[36] as it was an easy way to quantify the energy in all food.

However, as we will discuss further in this section, our bodies are a subtle interplay of systems, and so hitting it with the blunt instrument of artificial overall caloric restriction doesn't make much sense.

Conventional wisdom has an absolutist model of diet, based on the first law of thermodynamics:
"In a closed system, energy is always conserved"
which leads to "the equation of weight loss" being expressed as the very simple, elegant and utterly wrong
"calories in < calories out = weight loss"

---

[36]https://www.sciencedaily.com/releases/2006/11/0611 20060301.htm and
https://academic.oup.com/jn/article/136/12/2957/4663 943

In this model, the only way to "lose weight" is to create an energy deficit by restricting our energy intake to a level that is beneath the body's total energy output.

Because of the theories around heart health, it further states that carbohydrate should be the main food choice, as it carries less than half the calories of fat, a barely sufficient amount of protein to allow for body maintenance and it also states that consuming only limited supplies of calorie dense fat, and particularly saturated fats is the way to eat.

Finally, it dictates that having enough willpower to ignore hunger is paramount, and suffering hunger is normal and for your greater good.

However, what this model doesn't take account of is the second law of thermodynamics:
"Energy spontaneously disperses if it is not hindered."

This law is about energy dissipation; that no system is perfect, and that the tendency of all systems is to fall towards chaos (Entropy).

To quote Dr Michael Eades:[37]

"The second law of thermodynamics says that the entropy of the universe increases during any spontaneous process. What this means is that it is impossible for a system to turn a given amount of energy into an equivalent amount of work.

---

[37]https://proteinpower.com/drmike/2007/10/04/thermodynamics-and-weight-loss/

It is this second law that is really the 'a calorie is a calorie' law, and, in fact, the second law shows, in terms of weight loss at least, that a calorie isn't necessarily a calorie.

These two laws of thermodynamics can be summed up cleverly. The first law says you can't get something for nothing, and the second law tells you that you can't break even."

There is no system on earth, biological or manmade that uses 100% of the energy put in to create a 100% exact output. If there were, or could be, the much posited "perpetual motion machine" would be a thing, and we would all be living with free energy!

But no, perpetual motion cannot happen because of friction and heat – you must always put in slightly more energy than you will get out of the machine to keep it moving.

This begs the question, why does conventional wisdom think of the body as a "perfect machine" to have created the "calories in < calories out = weight loss" model? Scientific arrogance maybe? Possibly even a little Abrahamic religion leaking in to our science, as we are "made perfect in God's vison?" This is too much philosophy for me, but an interesting question none the less.

What the conventional model also doesn't take account of is that the body is not a bomb calorimeter, it does not literally "burn calories," rather it has various hormonal responses to the food we eat[38] and does not use all the food we eat as pure energy. Also, the various systems themselves leak energy, as all systems do, to a greater or lesser extent.

The body is a biological machine that has a rather large entropic tendency. When viewed in this light, calorie theory is a massive mis-interpretation of the 1st law of thermodynamics, with a total disregard of the 2nd law.

This is why with a low carb way of life, there is no need to make yourself a slave to a complex and limiting "calorie counting" regime as part of your life (unless you are the type of person that likes having the raw data of course!)

Another thing that kills off calorie theory is that beyond the actions of our hormones, our body treats the macronutrients very differently in terms of processing them to meet the body's needs.

---

[38]https://www.dietdoctor.com/first-law-thermodynamics-utterly-irrelevant

Carbohydrate

❖ Carbohydrate is used exclusively as an energy source by the body, either for burning straight away or converting into Glycogen for short term storage or Triglycerides, aka fat, for long-term storage. Note that conversion of glucose to triglycerides is a one-way process.

❖ Glucose enters the cell mitochondria, gets split up into 2 Pyruvate molecules which oxidise easily to form "Acetyl-Coenzyme A" which are then fed into the Krebs cycle[39] to produce adenosine triphosphate (ATP).

❖ ATP is the chemical that is oxidised by the body to provide energy.

○ I like to think of ATP as the body's "unit of energy currency", and the body's mitochondria as the "bureau de change" as it's the mitochondria that exchange glucose and ketones into ATP.

❖ Glucose exchange provides 38 ATP to the body.

❖ Glucose has no function in body repair at all beyond providing easy energy to drive the system.

❖ In terms of efficiency, carbohydrate is the least entropic and so the body favours it when it is available. In the presence of carbohydrate, all other potential sources of energy bar alcohol are ignored.

---

[39] The Krebs cycle (or citric acid cycle) is a part of cellular respiration. Named after Hans Krebs, it is a series of chemical reactions used by all aerobic organisms to generate energy from the food eaten.

Protein

❖ The body uses virtually all the protein we consume in the constant processes of body maintenance; your "soft" body structures are mostly made of protein and each no more than 2 weeks old. Even your bones, which are mostly calcified collagen, are only 10 years old at most. As well as building new cells and repairing old ones, we use protein to create hormones and enzymes. Protein also ensures the immune system stays optimal.

❖ Except when fasting, we need to eat a constant supply of high quality protein to power this renewal process, 0.5g per kg of lean body mass (the only place that "target weight" is useful) is a consumption minimum to ensure muscle and bone mass are preserved.

❖ If there is a protein deficiency in our diet, the body will slowly take protein from "non-essential systems" i.e. our muscles and bones, to repair our organs so that they remain in tip-top shape and we can keep living as long as possible.

❖ These healing and rebuilding processes dissipate some of our available energy and the body's protein use generates heat as a by-product which dissipates even more energy back to our environment.

❖ The body can convert protein into glucose via the process of gluconeogenesis that can then feed into the energy cycle in four situations, the first two being far more dire than the others:

1. Under semi-starvation conditions both consumed protein and body protein is converted into glucose to power the brain and heart. Semi-starvation is where only low nutrient density, mostly carbohydrate food is available.

2. Total starvation results in the body using its own protein as fodder for glucose conversion. Total starvation occurs after a very long time without food, when the body considers its fat reserves to be too low (the body maintains 7% body fat as it's absolute minimum) and will start rapidly consuming its protein to provide glucose instead of deriving ketones from fat.

3. If we consume an excess to repair requirement, the "leftover" protein can't simply sit around doing nothing, and so gets converted into glucose

4. If an organ requires glucose, and there is none readily available, protein is converted to serve the need. The kidneys in particular are glucose hungry, and really don't like running on ketones. They are a significant location where gluconeogenesis takes place, even when we are fully fat adapted[40]

---

[40] Berg JM, Tymoczko JL, Stryer L. Biochemistry. 5th edition. New York: W H Freeman; 2002. Section 30.2, Each Organ Has a Unique Metabolic Profile. Available from: https://www.ncbi.nlm.nih.gov/books/NBK22436/

- ❖ Fasting is not the same as starvation. In a fasted state, where no food is consumed for a short time and the body runs on ketones, protein is spared for recycling into the repair system, not converted into glucose.
- ❖ Most people eating the currently recommended low calorie/low fat diet eat less protein than the body requires to sustain itself healthily. This means that the increase to "protein adequate" that changing to a low carb way of life brings can feel like a "high protein diet." Where in fact, all it is giving the body is the right amount of building blocks for health.
- ❖ Also worth noting, the body's natural appetite regulation stops us eating too much protein – Protein eaten in excess of body need causes a nausea signal.
    - o Which is one very good reason why there is no need to count protein; if you are paying attention to the signals that your body is sending, unless you willingly choose to push past the signals, you cannot "over eat" protein.

Fat

- ❖ Only a portion of the fats we eat is available for converting into energy, as the body uses consumed cholesterol and other essential fatty acids to create hormones, cell walls and nerve sheathing (myelin).
- ❖ When the body works to convert fat into energy, it takes more intermediate steps than glucose,

first there is conversion into ketones, via β-oxidation of fatty acids, which can then become Acetyl-CoA which goes through the Krebs cycle to be exchanged into ATP.

❖ A ketone molecule exchanges for 129 ATP as opposed to the 38 ATP that glucose does[41].

   o As you can see, even though fat has just over twice the "calorie content" of protein and carbohydrate, it generates over three times the energy in the mitochondria!

❖ As with protein, the body's natural appetite regulation also stops us eating too much fat – fat eaten in excess of body need also causes a nausea signal.

Add to this the complicating fact that our gut microbiome also has an effect on the processing of all our food (which is so important it gets its own section) – The differences in microbiome means that if you feed the same plateful of food to a room full of people, they will all extract differing amounts of nutrients and energy from it.

All this all means that when eating a carbohydrate focused, barely protein adequate, low fat diet "the first law of thermodynamics is being upheld," as we are only burning glucose, which has no other body function bar becoming energy or fat. However, in these conditions, burning our own body fat is almost impossible.

_____

[41]http://cristivlad.com/energy-levels-under-ketosis-fats-carbs-and-atp/

It's only overnight when digestion has finished and the stomach is empty that levels of Insulin are ramped down to a point where fat burning to power overnight body maintenance can commence.

This means that weight reductions seen with low calorie, high carbohydrate dieting include a gradual muscle and bone wasting along with a fat reduction, due to our muscle protein being converted into glucose to provide energy. Muscle mass reduction leads to a reduction in the basal metabolic rate, which when a more usual level of calorie consumption is resumed results in a rebound fat gain, especially if you have the type of body that is pre-disposed to fatten easily[42].

Apart from the hunger, a common complaint from dieters faithfully sticking to this style of dieting is that they are always cold, for two reasons. Firstly, a ramped down metabolism doesn't expend as much heat as usual anyway, and if there is not quite enough protein being eaten anyway, the naturally thermogenic effect of eating it is missed.

Whist the laws of thermodynamics are what they are, and the basis of modern nutritional science is built around their seeming immutability, our bodies are biology, not physics. The "calorie theory" interpretation of the laws of thermodynamics bear no relation to how our bodies work.

---

[42]Richard MacKarness, Eat Fat and Grow Slim,1958: http://www.ourcivilisation.com/fat/chap1.htm

Given the very different amounts of actual energy we derive from our food as opposed to what a bomb calorimeter tells us they contain, and that we are not using all our food as pure energy, and that the various chemical processes that it takes to turn our food into either energy or parts of our body are wasteful processes, I trust that you will agree with me that "counting calories" is a pretty pointless exercise.

Yes, I know, you might be feeling very triggered right now, I've turned the whole hypothesis about how we are meant to eat on its head.

My "popping the bubble of calorie theory" may well cause you cognitive dissonance, as your mind struggles to see the facts through the stories you've always told yourself.

I suspect this is one reason why calorie theory has persisted as long as it has. Scientists hate cognitive dissonance, and when reading papers, it can be seen that many of the authors wilfully ignore biological facts so that the current theories can be maintained.

What are "Macronutrients" and how are they processed?

As I touched on in the last section, protein, carbohydrate and fat together are known as Macronutrients. The word itself is derived from the Greek *makros* mashed together with the Latin *nutriens* creating a word that has the meaning "food that nourishes." It first appears in Agriculture books in 1939, and then applying to food and diet in 1942.

The words protein and carbohydrate were invented in the 1840's to describe then new discoveries in chemistry about how the world works. Before then, protein wasn't described separately, and although we know now that there is some protein in most food, before the Victorians started scientifically investigating everything, "flesh" was probably the word that covered it best. As to carbohydrate, we described the two types separately, as "farinaceous (starch) and saccharine (sugar) matters."

Carbohydrate

Carbohydrate is a combination of the roots "carbo-" and "-hydrate"; this was because first observations pointed to carbohydrates being formed of a carbon atom binding to water molecules in a 2:1 ration - $C_m(H_2O)_n$ is the "cover all" formula used to express carbohydrate in science.

Hence, they were initially thought of as being "hydrates of carbon." This turned out not to be true, but by then the new scientific name had stuck.

As I said above, carbohydrates provide fuel to our cells. Apart from the monosaccharides ribose and xylose and of course fibre, that's their only job.

Carbohydrates come in three types; monosaccharides, disaccharides and polysaccharides.

There are 5 monosaccharides;

- ❖ Glucose (AKA dextrose - "right sugar")
- ❖ Fructose (AKA laevulose - "left sugar")
- ❖ Galactose
- ❖ Ribose
- ❖ Xylose

Glucose converts to ATP easily in all of our cells, but it doesn't do so all that efficiently. However, the body priorities ease over efficiency and as such, our bodies have evolved to always have some on hand; we have a strictly controlled amount of glucose running around in our blood and also have stores of glucose as the polysaccharide glycogen that can easily convert back to glucose to fuel the cells as required.

Because glucose is so important to all life, we can also make our own glucose from protein, by the process of gluconeogenesis. Gluconeogenesis is why there is no biological need to eat any carbohydrate at all.

80% of the glucose we eat heads off to hang out in our blood, where Insulin ushers it into our cells; either our muscles and organs to create ATP to power the body or into fats cells to be stored. The other 20% heads down to the liver where it mostly it turned into glycogen for later use, which is a good and healthy thing and has kept us alive for millennia. When runner's carb load with pasta, this glycogen storage mechanism is what they are taking advantage of so that they have energy for the run.

A tiny amount of the glucose consumed turns into pyruvate, which heads through the Krebs cycle, turns into citrate which then becomes a lipid droplet that is then encased in the very low density lipoprotein (VLDL) type of cholesterol. VLDL is the lipoprotein that transports these lipid droplets and transported away to our visceral fat cells.

Both this de novo lipogenesis process and the glycogen repletion cycle tells the pancreas to calm down and taper off Insulin response, which tells the brain that it doesn't need any more food.

High levels of VLDL in the blood is now well established as the main cause of arterial plaque. However, the amount of glucose that gets turned into VLDL is tiny, around 1/50th of any glucose consumed. So, in the big picture, glucose becoming VLDL isn't really the issue to our overall health.

Glucose forms long chains easily and so is the building block for all the polysaccharides, AKA digestible complex carbs and indigestible fibre. As omnivores, our bodies produce an enzyme (amylase) to break apart the polysaccharides we lump together as starches, but not the enzyme (cellulase) to break apart fibre.

Galactose bonds together with glucose to make the disaccharide lactose, found in milk, which only around 35% of the humans on the planet can digest after weening. Galactose is processed via the same pathways as glucose, so is metabolically nigh on identical to glucose.

Ribose is rather fascinating in its own way. We don't use it for energy at all, instead, our bodies make ribose as an essential to life molecule. It is the backbone of DNA, RNA, and ATP.

We can boost our production of ribose by eating Vitamin B2 (riboflavin) rich food. [43]
It's also found in small amount in
- ❖ Mushrooms
- ❖ Beef and poultry
- ❖ Cheddar cheese and cream cheese
- ❖ Milk
- ❖ Eggs
- ❖ Caviar
- ❖ Anchovies, herring, and sardines
- ❖ Yoghurt

Recently, d-ribose supplementation at doses way more than we would ever consume naturally have been studied. Study participants took 3x5g per day, and the early research show benefits for patients with chronic heart failure (CHF), improving muscle stamina and regulating blood circulation in the heart[44]. It's also been

---

[43]https://en.wikibooks.org/wiki/Structural_Biochemistry/Nucleic_Acid/Sugars/Ribose
[44] http://www.nutridesk.com.au/simple-sugars.phtml

shown to cause pain reduction for patients with fibromyalgia.[45]

Xylose is "wood sugar" and so, as we don't eat trees, it is not in human food at all. We discovered its relative xylitol in the late 19th century, and we started wholesale manufacture in the 1970's because it was seen to have a protective effect on teeth. Xylitol wrecks our microbiome however, as I discussed earlier.

Fructose and Ethanol

As fructose is a monosaccharide and ethanol is a hydrocarbon, a carbohydrate of a slightly different shape, neither are classed officially as a macronutrient. However, the body processes both of them via their own separate, very similar, pathway. So, they deserve a section to themselves.

Fructose is more commonly known as "fruit sugar" as it is found in fruit, vegetables and honey. Long chains of fructose have their own special name, fructans, which are found in certain vegetables, wheat and other cereal grains and fruit.

Sucrose (what we call sugar) is a disaccharide made from glucose and fructose bonding together. Fructose is the part that makes sucrose sweet to our taste buds. Glucose on its own is 0.8 times less sweet than sugar,

---

[45]https://www.drweil.com/vitamins-supplements-herbs/supplements-remedies/does-ribose-really-energize/

whereas fructose on its own is 1.17 times sweeter than sugar.

In the US, the corporate search for cheaper sugar sources that could allow cheaper production of low fat foods led to the invention of "High Fructose Corn Syrup" (HFCS) which is 45% glucose and 55% Fructose.

HFCS is made from "yellow #2 dent corn", a crop engineered to feed cows, not humans. Dent corn carries a heavy US government subsidy, making it far cheaper to grow than sugar cane or sugar beet.

As sucrose breaks down in the body immediately into glucose and fructose, this led manufacturers and the USDA to consider HFCS synonymous with sucrose in food use, even though it is a touch sweeter.

Thankfully, we don't have HFCS in any of our UK foods, as we have a thriving sugar processing industry which imports sugar cane from commonwealth countries and then exports sugar to all of Europe! However, we do have "invert sugar" in some of our baked goods and confectionary - a solution of sucrose heated with either citric acid or enzymes to split apart the sucrose molecule to produce a sweeter and more stable solution.

So, why is artificially separating the glucose and fructose, and having a solution that is richer in fructose than would be natural a problem? For that matter, what's the problem with eating sucrose?

It's because, as I mentioned above, in the body enzymes split sucrose into a molecule of glucose and a molecule of fructose, the very reason why the USDA see HFCS as synonymous with sucrose.

In its natural form, fructose is bound to fibre in fruit, or is provided in small, seasonal amounts as honey or maple syrup. Fructose is nature's way of fattening us up for winter. There are also no easily edible by human sources of available sucrose that do not have masses of fibre included.

We have to process the very fibrous sugar cane or sugar beet to get at sucrose in quantity, meaning that until around 120 years ago, pure sucrose was rare and expensive in the human diet.

Fructose has its own metabolic pathways and unlike glucose, which the whole body can metabolise, fructose is treated as a poison and wholly metabolised by the liver.

100% of the fructose consumed turns into acetate which goes through the Krebs cycle just like pyruvate to eventually becomes lipid droplets encased in VLDL as well as some free fatty acids, which head out to muscles to find a home (causing muscle-based Insulin resistance as a side issue) via *de novo* lipogenesis. It also produces a little bit of uric acid as a metabolite by-product, which in large amounts causes gout and hypertension.

If you eat more fructose than the liver can handle, the lipid droplets don't get wrapped up safely in VLDL for transport, instead they get stuck in your liver, leading to

Non-Alcoholic Related Fatty Liver Disease (NAFLD) and its more serious cousins; Non-alcohol Related Steatohepatitis (NASH), NASH with fibrosis and ultimately cirrhosis.

Fructose consumption also causes inflammation of the liver by activating the "JNK1" enzyme which causes liver-based Insulin resistance, which makes the pancreas produce more Insulin (hyperinsulinemia) which negates Leptin's action on the brain.

When eating in its natural state, fructose is buffered with fibre that fills us up and stops us consuming more than our body can handle in a sitting.

However, the current craze for smoothies, juices and fibre stripped foods means that the liver can be easily overwhelmed by an unnatural tsunami of fructose. There is no way you could eat 4 applies in one sitting, but it's easy to drink 4 apple's worth of juice in one go.

Fructose also doesn't suppress Ghrelin production in the gut like glucose does – you can consume fibreless fructose or sucrose containing products until you are literally bursting and stay ravenously hungry. Fructose and sucrose are intensely unsatiating substances.

Fructose doesn't stimulate Insulin or Leptin either – which is why fructose has been "seen as good for people with diabetes", as it doesn't cause an Insulin surge. I trust you agree with me that what it does in the body is far worse!

So, what does fructose have in common with alcohol? And here I'm talking specifically about ethanol, the only non-instantly toxic alcohol to the human body.

The brain and stomach process 20% of the ethanol between them, which is us getting drunk and is also why ethanol is considered an "acute toxin" in excess.

The remaining 80% heads off to the liver where it breaks down into acetaldehyde (which as an aside directly contributes to cirrhosis by damaging liver proteins), which then turns into acetate and then goes through the same processing pathway as fructose. The other by-products are reactive oxygen species (ROS), which again damage proteins in the liver.

If you drink more ethanol than the liver can handle, the triglycerides build up get stuck in there, leading to Fatty Liver Disease, Alcohol Related Steatohepatitis (ASH), ASH with Fibroids and Cirrhosis.

As I mentioned in the introduction, Dr Robert Lustig explains the glucose, fructose and ethanol pathways with pretty diagrams in his "Sugar: The bitter truth" lecture - If you love this geeky stuff, this link skips to 42:20 so you can see all the biochemistry.
https://youtu.be/dBnniua6-oM?t=42m20s

So, as fructose and ethanol turn directly into visceral body fat, eating a diet high in fructose and/or ethanol is essentially a highly and dangerously fattening diet.

Dr Lustig also postulates that because we eat and drink way more fructose now than we have ever done (especially as children are now given fizzy drinks and juice rather than water, and also in hot countries that drink no alcohol at all but are consuming sugared carbonated beverages like they are going out of fashion) this is leading to the massive upswing in incidence of NAFLD, which is the first step in the body towards Insulin resistance.

It's been shown that Insulin resistance is the cause of Metabolic Syndrome AKA Syndrome X –"abnormal cholesterol, high blood pressure and high blood glucose leading to diabetes and/or visceral obesity" – a syndrome that a great deal of the "civilised world" population now have.

Protein

Protein comes from the Greek linguistic roots *proteios* "the first quality," and it starts appearing in scientific literature around the 1840s.

Protein is the major building block for all of our body structures and contains 11 nonessential amino acids and 9 essential amino acids – these essential amino acids are substances that we need to live, thrive and survive, and that we cannot manufacture for ourselves. We have to consume the 9 essential amino acids from the food we eat.

The nonessential amino acids can be made by the body; however you must have all of the amino acids in order that your body can maintain the wide variety of structures of which it's made. [46]

When we ingest protein, the body breaks it down into its constituent amino acids and then it wants to use them exclusively for body repair. As body repair is of vital importance for life, the body only uses protein to make ATP under duress, via converting protein to glucose via gluconeogenesis.

Another important point to note is that the hormone Cortisol inhibits amino acid synthesis.[47] Whilst that's not a problem if we live a non-stressful lifestyle, the pace of modern life rarely allows for this. We over produce Cortisol when under prolonged stress, which leads to a whole host of other issues I've already covered.

Fat

The word fat has been used in literature since at least the 1500's, which is as far back as I can casually search for it via Google Ngrams, and it comes with a whole tonne of accompanying baggage.

It came into Modern English via Old English *fǣtt* "well fed, fatted, plump" which was originally a contracted past participle of *fǣttian* "to cram, stuff full"

---

[46] https://en.wikipedia.org/wiki/Amino_acid_synthesis
[47] Manchester KL (1964). "Sites of Hormonal Regulation of Protein Metabolism". In Munro HN, Allison JB. Mammalian protein metabolism. 4. New York: Academic Press. p. 229 - ISBN 978-0-12-510604-7.

It's not all bad however, it also come from Proto-Indo-European as a very positive and abundant word: from the root *peie-* "to be fat, swell" comes *poid-* "to abound in water, milk, fat, etc." itself sourced from a mash up of Greek *piduein* "to gush forth" and Sanskrit *payate* "swells, exuberates" and *pituh* "juice, sap, resin"

Also throw in some Greek *pion* "fat; wealthy" and the Latin *pinguis* "fat"; and you can see that the word Fat has carried many many meanings ever since language evolved.

Until very recently, dietary fat sources have been celebrated rather than vilified. Hunter gatherer tribes will eat the fat and brains of an animal before the lean muscle and organ meats, and even up to the early part of the 20th century, a diet higher in fat and lower in sugars and starches was considered healthful.

For instance Dr Benjamin Spock, in his book "The Common Sense Book of Baby and Child care", published in 1946: *'Rich desserts can be omitted without risk, and should be, by anyone who is obese and trying to reduce. The amount of plain, starchy foods (cereals, breads, potatoes) taken is what determines, in the case of most people, how much (weight) they gain or lose"*

In the early 19th Century, Jean Anthelme Brillat-Savarin[48] claimed that he could easily identify the cause of obesity; after thirty years of talking with obese people that

---

[48] https://en.wikipedia.org/wiki/Jean_Anthelme_Brillat-Savarin

proclaimed the joys of bread, rice, and potatoes to him, it was obvious to him that this was the issue. His recommended reducing diet, not surprisingly, was *'more or less rigid abstinence from everything that is starchy or floury."*

There are three types of fat, all of which contain a range of "essential fatty acids"

- ❖ Saturated
- ❖ Monounsaturated
- ❖ Polyunsaturated

And fat containing foods provide these fats in various ratios:

- ❖ Animal fats are composed of mostly saturated and monounsaturated fats, with a small amount of polyunsaturated fats
- ❖ Marine fats are mostly monounsaturated and polyunsaturated with a lesser amount of saturated fats.
- ❖ Plant fats are composed of monounsaturated fats and polyunsaturated fats in varying ratios.
  - o The notable exceptions are Coconut and Palm oil. Coconut oil is almost entirely saturated fat, whereas palm oil has the same sort of fat profile as animal fat.

The "Lipid Hypothesis"

"Saturated fats cause Chronic Heart Disease" was first posited in the 1950's by Ancel Keys and is now widely accepted as truth by most western governments.

However, this hypothesis has no actual scientific evidence that proves it to be true in humans, despite 60 years of trials trying to provide this proof.

Amongst other things, the hypothesis has given us guidance to move away from saturated fat and towards polyunsaturated fats, which in excess are utterly terrible for our bodies.

Linoleic acid, the major polyunsaturated fatty acid found in vegetable oils is an essential fatty acid, but we only need a small amount for our health. Large amounts of polyunsaturated fats (PUF) in general and linoleic acid in particular are an immune system suppressant.

The first person to suggest that polyunsaturated fats suppress the immune system was Dr R A Newsholme of Oxford University in 1977[49]. What Newsholme wrote was that when our diet is rich and includes a plentiful amount of PUF, the immunosuppressive power of PUF make us prone to infection by bacteria and viruses.

He was making the point that the immunosuppressive effects of PUFs in sunflower seeds could be useful in treating autoimmune diseases such as multiple sclerosis[50] and that the same fatty acids could also be used to suppress the immune system to prevent rejection of kidney transplants, which due to medical

---

[49] Newsholme E A. Mechanism for starvation suppression and refeeding activity of infection. *Lancet* 1977; i: 654.

[50] Miller JD, *et al.Br Med J* 1973; i: 765.

advances at that time were just becoming a real possibility.

Newsholme posited that there was no better way to immunosuppress a renal patient than with sunflower seed oil, which is rich in linoleic acid.

Doctors using Newsholme's proposed protocol discovered that it effectively prevented kidney rejection but kicked up the incidence of all cancers; by twenty times over the expected norm for some cancers

Which logically is to be expected, as anything that suppresses the immune system over time is likely to cause cancer.

The findings around cancer were also in line with heart studies using diets that were high in PUFs which, reported an excess of cancer deaths from as early as 1971[51]

In 1989 there was a report of a ten-year heart study trial at a Veterans' Administration Hospital in Los Angeles. In this trial half the patients were given a diet which had double the amount of PUFs as compared to saturated fat (SF)

There was a fifteen percent increase in cancer deaths in the half of the patients in the high PUF group compared to the control group[52].

---

[51] Pearce M L, Dayton S. Incidence of cancer in men on a diet high in polyunsaturated fat. *Lancet* 1971; i: 464.

[52] American Heart Association Monograph, No 25.*1969.*

The authors of the report stated that the PUFs had been the cause of the increase in cancer deaths.

In 1991, two studies, from USA[53] and Canada[54], specifically found that linoleic acid increased the risk of breast tumours. Experiments with a variety of fats showed that saturated fats did not cause tumours but, when small amounts of polyunsaturated oil or pure linoleic acid were added to the diet, this greatly increased the incidence of breast cancer.

All of the above is why I grade seed oils as non-optimal on the OSN scale, and suggests why Professor Noakes put them on his "Banting Red List." in Real Meal Revolution.

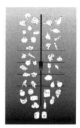

The bad news doesn't stop there though...

Omega 6 vs Omega 3

As well as Linoleic acid, the other body negative thing to come out of the guidance to move away from saturated fat and towards polyunsaturated fats is the shift in the ratio of Omega 6 to Omega 3 essentials polyunsaturated fatty acids (PUFA).

---

[53] Carroll K K. Dietary fats and cancer. Am J Clin Nutr 1991; 53: 1064S.

[54] France T, Brown P. Test-tube cancers raise doubts over fats. New Scientist, 7 December 1991, p 12.

Studies suggest that in our past, our diets contained around a 1:1 ratio of Omega 6 to Omega 3 PUFA. The Modern Western Diet contains a ratio that is more like 15:1.

Omega 6 PUFA are inflammatory, and Omega 3 PUFA anti-inflammatory. In balance, both PUFA serve us, but out of balance, the inflammatory properties of Omega 6 increase underlying factors for chronic disease.

Chronic inflammation has been shown to increase the risk factors for cancer, arterial sclerosis, coronary heart disease, chronic obstructive pulmonary disease (COPD), gut issues such as inflammatory bowel syndrome (IBS) and Chron's, and the inflammatory arthritis types such as rheumatoid and psoriatic.

Inflammation also interferes with sleep and is currently being investigated as the root cause of depression and is thought to be a factor towards increased Insulin resistance.[55]

I'm sure that you will agree with me that immunosuppression and inflammation aren't desirable.

Putting our Omega 6 to Omega 3 ratio back to a more natural 1:1 is a simple matter of reducing our plant oil consumption to nigh on zero whilst maintaining consumption of naturally rich Omega 3 sources, such as

---

[55]http://www.health.com/health/gallery/0,,20898778,0 0.html

oily fish, free range eggs, nuts and the fat of well reared meat.

Our increased consumption of Seed oils is another case where science is "sticking its fingers in its ears and going 'la-la-la!'" and causing us to medicate our way around the issues. Removing seed oils is a very simple way of redressing the balance back to where out bodies expect our fatty acid profile intake to be.

Micronutrients – AKA Vitamins and minerals

So, we've talked about the macronutrients, let's get into talking about the micronutrients. Micronutrients are all the other substances that our body needs to live thrive and survive, beyond protein, fat and carbohydrate. Deficiencies in these substances cause serious issues, such as beriberi, rickets, pellagra and scurvy.

The argument that the best way to consume all of the vitamins and minerals required for health is via our food is based upon a "cure of deficiency to prevent sickness" model. The research performed back in the 1930's and 40's into the effect of vitamins and minerals on the body was all based around curing deficiency, finding a minimum required level to not be sick, which became what we now know as the "Nutrient Reference Value"[56] and that is where science and research stopped.

Beyond curing disease, academia saw no more need to pursue the subject. So much so, that when Oxford University were offered a large endowment to conduct nutritional research into micronutrients, they turned it down, with the attitude of "We've already identified all the essential nutrients. What more is there to do?"[57]

---

[56] Before 2014, it was the "Recommended Daily Allowance" https://www.justvitamins.co.uk/blog/rda-or-nrv/

[57] Dr Atkins' Vita-Nutrient Solution, Fireside Edition 1999, Pg 26. ISBN 0-684-84488-5

Whilst it's worth the consideration that our bodies are better able to digest the vitamins and minerals that comes from food, as bio-available sources that we have evolved to so easily utilise over millennia are always a good thing, we also now live in an era of far more intense farming than ever before in history with the use of unbalanced chemical rather than organic fertilisers.

This can lead to imbalance in our food's micronutrient makeup that our ancestors would never have seen.

So, whilst it's just about possible to prevent deficiency with our food, if you want to obtain micronutrients in doses that not only cure deficiency, but also optimise their effects in our body, high-quality supplementation is the way to go.

When I read books on this back in the early 2000's, I was shocked that many vitamins and minerals have as good or better effects when used in a targeted way as pharmaceuticals deployed to treat the same illnesses.

Luckily, not all scientists took the same attitude as Oxford, and there have been many studies showing that micronutrients, AKA "nutraceuticals", can have the same or better effects on the body as pharmaceuticals.

So, the first time around I took a multitude of supplements, that when I picked back up again in 2010, I forgot about why I took, only really remembering just how many pills it was and how expensive it could be!

However, as I've got back into the swing of things in the last two years or so, and also re-read the books I read on vitamins and minerals, I'm again a dedicated supplement taker.

The supplement industry is huge, in the UK it was worth an estimated £421,000,000 in 2016, and I personally think this is with good reason.

If you want to dive deep into this, I highly recommend reading "Dr Atkins' Vita-Nutrient solution" - https://amzn.to/2IgSXhj - a book that I think serves the world in an even better and deeper way than his diet books do – and with micronutrients, I highly do recommend doing your research. Stepping into taking supplements is not something to be done casually or with a scattergun approach.

For some of micronutrients, an overdose is as or more harmful than an underdose. For instance, iron comes in two forms, "heme" and "non-heme."

Heme indicates that the iron molecule is bound to haemoglobin, and so came from an animal source. Non-heme iron comes from plants and is much less well absorbed by the body.

Iron is also minimally excreted, most of the iron we eat stays with us, The only way to get rid of it is via blood loss, and so any "free iron" running around the body not bound to haemoglobin builds up in tissue, converting between ferrous and ferric states, causing oxidation damage.

High levels of iron are associated with higher risk of CHD, and it's been shown that menstruation, and so iron loss, is a huge protective against CHD in women of child-bearing age[58]

It's for this reason that I take a multi-vitamin and mineral that has no iron in it, and I also semi-regularly go and give blood.

Everyone's supplement regime will be a matter of individual need. However, there are some things that I believe everyone would benefit from.

If I were to name three micronutrients I consider essential, they would be Vitamin D, Omega 3 and Magnesium.

Vitamin D

In the UK, we simply don't get enough sun for most of the year, so we tend to run a little short of this vital hormone (yes, vitamin D is a hormone!) during winter. Vitamin D is not only used to help build our bones, its function is intertwined with most of our body systems.

Having optimal levels of D running around helps keep our skin healthy, allows the body to use calcium and magnesium to better effect when rebuilding nerves, aids blood glucose control, lowers blood pressure, helps the

---

[58]https://www.sciencedirect.com/science/article/pii/S01
40673681924636 and
https://academic.oup.com/ajcn/article/76/3/501/46774
13

bowel do its thing, reduces arthritic pain, boosts the immune system, decreases fatigue and even aids recovery from most cancers.[59]

Taking between 400IU and 800IU a day of vitamin D_3 during the winter is, I believe, a must. Ramp it down May-September, over the summer months, as four months of exposing your bare face and arms to outdoor sunlight for twenty minutes a day does the same, moneysaving, job as the supplementation in light skinned people.

Darker skinned people will either need more sun, or a constant lower level of supplementation during summer. One of the other reasons we can be D deficient is use of sunscreen, so enjoy that sun, get some free vitamin D and then be sun-wise to prevent burning.

Do not take more than 800IU regularly without medical supervision, as this is one of the micronutrients where "too much of a good thing" is detrimental to health. Too much vitamin D can lead to hypercalcemia, a build-up of calcium in the blood which can cause nausea and vomiting, weakness, constipation, confusion, abnormal heart rhythm and frequent urination.

---

[59] Although we cannot say "Vitamin D is cancer protective", in the lab it stops tumours growing, and there is an inverse relationship between sunlight and breast cancer incidence – Lefkowitz, E et al., International Journal of Epidemiology, 1994; 23(6): 1133-36

Always err on the side of caution with vitamin D unless you are under medical supervision for a recognised vitamin D deficiency.

Omega 3

The Omega 3 family of essential fatty acids contain three acids of note. Alpha-Linolenic Acid, (ALA) found in linseed (usually sold as flaxseed) oil, Eicosapentaenoic Acid (EPA) and Docosahexaenoic Acid (DHA) both found in cold-water fish oils.

As I mentioned above, the Omega 3's are extraordinarily anti-inflammatory! This reason alone is a good reason to supplement as all this anti-inflammatory action leads to a monumental amount of healing in the body.

They've been shown to massively increase heart health, lower the amount of low density lipoprotein (LDL) in the blood, lower blood pressure, reduce platelet clumping without impeding blood clotting factors, help to prevent cancer, "oil" our joints, boost the immune system, lung and kidney function, decrease fatigue and alleviate mood disorders.

Taking a good quality supplement is essential; these fats are quick to oxidize and deteriorate rapidly when exposed to sunlight. If you are buying free flowing oil rather than capsules, it must be refrigerated and in an opaque bottle. If it's not on display in the fridge of the shop you purchase it from, shop elsewhere.

Omega oil blends are popular and are also usually vegetarian. ALA can convert to DHA and EPA in the body, but it can take months for the levels to build to therapeutic levels, so, unless you have ethical reasons not to take animal oils, it's quicker to take 500-1000mg of both a high-quality Flaxseed oil and Fish oil daily.

Also note, taking vitamin E with DHA and EPA prevents them oxidizing, so check supplement ingredients; if it has at least 12mg of vitamin E included, (which is 100% NRV) this stops the oil going rancid in the capsule, but not enough to stop oxidation in the body.

Again, caution is advised, too much fish oil with no Vitamin E to prevent its deterioration causes oxidative damage to the body. Add in 400IU (268mg) of vitamin E per 1000mg of fish oil to keep this effect in check.

If you are suffering from an active inflammatory disease, such as asthma or arthritis, taking 3000-4000mg of good quality fish oil, along with 400IU of vitamin E and at least 1000mg of Vitamin C, spilt into three doses over around three months will go a long way to reducing the inflammation and so your symptoms and pain levels. Building up your stores of DHA and EPA over time and keeping them high is essential for remaining healthy.

Magnesium

Magnesium (Mg) is the most important mineral for heart health. It keeps our tickers beating steadily, smoothing out arrythmia, it relaxes constricted blood vessels, allowing blood to flow more freely, lowering blood pressure and reducing angina, as well as preventing platelets from clumping, which means that the blood is less likely to form artery blocking clots.

Also, more than 300 enzymes depend on a steady supply of Mg for their production, Mg helps keep potassium (K) in balance as they work together antagonising sodium (Na) and calcium (Ca) mediating water flow in and out of cells, as well as keeping Ca in our bones where it should be rather than being excreted.

It helps to stabilise blood glucose levels, decreases mood swings with PMT (which is the reason that women crave chocolate just before their period, as cocoa mass is a potent Mg delivery system), enables muscles to grow effectively, encourages bronchial muscles to relax (an IV push of Mg stops an asthma attack cold) as well as helping to alleviate migraines, potentially by relaxing the muscles that are cutting blood supply off to the brain (studies have found that regular intake of magnesium reduced the frequency of migraine attacks by around 40% percent[60]) and yet most of us are deficient in Mg.

---

[60] Sun-Edelstein C, Mauskop A. Alternative headache treatments: nutraceuticals, behavioral and physical treatments. Headache. 2011 Feb;51(3):469-483. https://doi.org/10.1111/j.1526-4610.2011.01846.x

Mauskop A, Altura BT, et al. Intravenous magnesium sulphate relieves migraine attacks in patients with low serum ionized magnesium levels: a pilot study. Clin Sci (Lond). 1995 Dec;89(6):633-6.

The standard diet is also woefully short of Mg, as many of the foods that contain it are either being grown in mineral deficient soil, or in food that some people are not wild about anyway (leafy greens) or in food that is frowned upon as containing fat. (avocado, high quality dark chocolate, egg yolk, nuts and seeds)

Happily, leafy greens, nuts, seeds, high quality dark chocolate, avocado and egg yolks are the stalwarts of a low carb way of eating. However, you may also find that you simply feel better with Mg supplementation also.

NB: if you have a kidney issue, you must have careful medical supervision if you are thinking of upping your Mg.

Taking 200mg of Magnesium a day hits the spot nicely. Or, take an Epsom salt bath. Add 500g of Epsom salt to a warm bath and soak for 15 minutes, two or three times a week. Your body will absorb what it needs through your skin, no muss, no fuss.

Micronutrient "insurance"

Aside from the "top three" I feel that if you can do nothing more, aside from eating real food, the best source of micronutrients there is, a good quality multi-vitamin and mineral offers a nice all-round bump. I personally take Holland and Barrett "ABC plus seniors" as it has good all-round coverage, and no iron in it to cause free radical damage.

My advice here is to do your own research, have a read of supplement labels, and get the best all-rounder without iron that you can afford.

I'd also highly recommend reading further books on nutraceuticals if you are interested in delving further into this subject. It's a rather fascinating field of study.

What does this all mean for the "UK healthy diet" we've been told to eat?

Before 1983 there were no overarching public health nutrition guidelines, and there had been no 'food policy' since World War II. The UK establishment very much felt that fat was not a health problem and carbs made you fat.

The Nutrition Advisory Committee on Nutrition Education (NACNE) chaired by Philip James, authored a paper[61] that set out consumption guidance on amounts of fat, salt, sugar and fibre for the UK population.

The paper generally got on board with the hypothesis of Ancel Key's around saturated fats, and apart from anything else the committee noted that *'The previous nutritional advice in the UK to limit the intake of all carbohydrates as a means of weight control now runs counter to current thinking and contrary to the present proposals for a nutrition education policy for the population as a whole... The problem then becomes one of achieving both a reduction in fat intake to 30% of total energy and a fall in saturated fatty acid intake to 10%"*

So, when I went looking for the stats for this book I expected that the UK would mirror the US in its climbing

[61] "A Discussion Paper on Proposals for Nutritional Guidelines for Health Education in Britain."
National Advisory Committee on Nutrition Education (1983) London: Health Education Council.

sugar consumption as manufacturers scrambled to replace fats with sugar in "low-fat products" for taste reason.

Imagine my surprise when I saw graphs that showed this not to be the case! Our sugar consumption has been gently falling for the last forty years, whilst the US consumption has been skyrocketing.[62] [63]

So, I went digging further, and discovered the below graph, in a blog post written with the opinion that as "we've dropped sugar consumption, we can't blame "Big Sugar" for the rise of our obesity problem. Everyone just needs to exercise more!"[64] The same old hideous refrain "Fat people are greedy and lazy, it's their own fault they're fat"

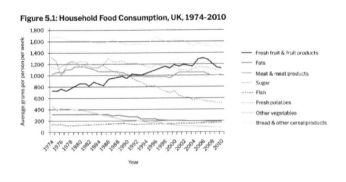

Figure 5.1: Household Food Consumption, UK, 1974-2010

[62] https://plot.ly/~vizthinker/19/sugar-consumption-us-canada-eu/

[63] https://plot.ly/~vizthinker/27/average-bmi-us-canada-eu/

[64] http://theviewfromcullingworth.blogspot.co.uk/2013/08/sugar-more-from-new-puritans.html

Looking at this graph, I saw that since 1974, we've dropped our added sugar consumption from over 450g per week to around 90g in 2010. For unknown reasons we've also dropped the amount of potatoes we eat from around 1.3Kg a week to around 500g as well as dropping our total fat consumption from 300g to 200g per week.

The amount of bread per week has dropped slightly, from around 1.7Kg to 1.3Kg whilst Meat, Fish and "other vegetables" have stayed roughly the same – 1Kg, 160g, 1.1Kg per week respectively.

The big climber on this chart is "Fruit and Fruit products" – we've gone from around 750g per week to a whopping peak of 1.3Kg per week in 2006, with a slight drop to around 1.15Kg per week in 2010.

Fruit Products included fruit juice, which of course is an unbuffered source of pure fructose.

And when my brain figured out what I was looking at, I literally exclaimed out loud "It's the fructose… It's the fructose!"

Now, we all know that statistics prove that statistics prove nothing. In particular, the link that the 'blog references about where they got the graph from does not lead directly back to how the graph was generated, and as I do so love primary source data and being right, I was initially loath to use it as a reference source.

So I dug about a bit more and discovered that the above graph is based on the "Family Food Open Data" which is a yearly survey of half a million British families' eating habits[65] Interestingly, I found graphs from the same data set in the Daily Mail, showing that our consumption of Rice, Pasta, Pizza increased as our consumption of potatoes has decreased, although spuds are by far still our most popular "starchy side" [66]

The Daily Mail graphs also show that our banana consumption has skyrocketed in the last 25 years, from around 80g per week before 1986 up to a whopping 220g in 2010, with a peak in 2006 of around 230g per week, matching the "fruit and fruit products" peaks in the first graph I found.

So, in the UK I feel we have a different reason for our obesity epidemic to the US. Whilst our current guidance originates from similar guidance in the US, I suspect that in the nation's efforts to "get healthy," we've very effectively cut down on the things that we've been told are harmful to health.

However, we've also upped the intake of something viewed as beneficial but is instead the very thing which is most harmful to our bodies in quantity, especially when fibre is removed from it.

---

[65]   https://www.gov.uk/government/collections/family-food-statistics

[66]http://www.dailymail.co.uk/news/article-3300658/Tinned-spaghetti-hoops-white-bread-potatoes-menu-British-families-culinary-dark-ages.html

I would posit that our decreased fat consumption, massively increased fructose consumption and continuous high levels of bread consumption is what is currently doing most of the harm to our nation's health.

I know that this opinion will be contentious, as a great deal of people very much enjoy eating high sugar fruits and fruit juices. However, as fructose is directly fattening, and this is where the UK has made its biggest caloric increase, I personally can draw no other conclusions from the data.

Intermittent fasting

As I'm writing this book, there is a great deal of buzz around intermittent fasting (IF) used in conjunction with a low carbohydrate way of eating on the internet. So, writing a section all about it seems appropriate.

It is in no way obligatory to do intermittent fasting when you are eating a low carbohydrate diet, however, many people seem to fall into a pattern of "skipping meals every now and then", simply because they are not hungry and following the second tenet. This can then develop naturally into a way of eating that has a large fasting window and so their way of life includes IF effortlessly.

There is a long tradition of fasting in various forms within many world religions[67]. Religious leaders of the past recognised that periods without food were restorative to the body and mind and appeared to bring fasting people closer to their spirituality. There is naturally more focus on regular fasting in the religions that seek to control and discipline the body, seeing it as a distraction towards Godliness.

In a physiological context, fasting refers to the metabolic status of a person who has not eaten for around 8 hours, for instance, overnight, or to the metabolic state achieved after complete digestion and absorption of a meal.

---

[67] https://en.wikipedia.org/wiki/Fasting#Religious_views

Fasting stimulates various body systems that promote fat burning, healing and growth, and so we can use this to our advantage as a tool to nudge along our progress to an optimal body.

It is worth noting however that the sexes react differently to it. The male body deals well with IF at any age, however, the female body and its constant roil of hormones can react to IF in the same way as it reacts to stress, meaning it can raise Cortisol levels and so inhibit fat burning.

However, in women over 45, as perimenopause kicks in, and the balance of hormones shift around, IF has been shown to be an effective tool to use against the "middle aged middle" that forms at this time, where Oestrogen production is ramping down and circulating follicle-stimulating hormone (FSH) rises to try and stimulate more Oestrogen production from our ovaries. The body then fights to keep Oestrogen where it was, and increasingly turns to our fat cells to make Oestrogen, hence making storing more fat a more valuable proposition to the body than it was previously.

How much Insulin we have running around also drives the action of Oestrogen, and Insulin production is extremely well regulated when fasting. So, as well as the hormone balancing and normalising benefits of eating a low carbohydrate diet anyway, this is the main reason why I recommend to all my female clients over 45 to give IF a bash as well as low carb eating and see how they go with it and how it makes them feel.

So, apart from the effect on Insulin, are there other reasons to fast?

Well, as Hippocrates allegedly said *"Our food should be our medicine, and medicine should be our food. However, to eat when we are sick, is to feed our sickness"*

He's talking about a "fasting instinct" – when we are ill, we don't really want to eat! The body knows that in a fasted state, it doesn't have to concentrate on digestion and so we heal more efficiently.

Whatever macronutrients our body is used to obtaining its energy from, when we are in a fasted state the body uses ketosis to power itself. When Insulin production reaches a natural low point from being in a fasted state, the healing process called Autophagy is stimulated.

Autophagy was discovered in the 1960's and documented by Yoshinori Ohsumi in 1992. His work is considered so important to our body of scientific knowledge that on October 3rd 2016, the Nobel Assembly at Karolinska Institutet awarded the Nobel Prize in Physiology or Medicine to him for his discoveries. [68]

The word autophagy originates from the Greek words auto-, meaning "self", and phagein, meaning "to eat". It's the natural way that the body cleans our cells of old,

_____

[68]https://www.nobelprize.org/nobel_prizes/medicine/laureates/2016/press.html

damaged and degraded matter, infectious agents and very efficiently recycles what it can to form new cells.

Autophagy helps us in many ways, but the "Insulin stimulating diet coupled with eating late and a sleep window of only 6-7 hours" pattern that is modern life, along with our generally regular daily eating of food doesn't allow this body process to really shine and do its job of healing us as effectively as it could do.

By extending the window in which overnight ketosis and autophagy operates, we give the body a much better window in which it can perform repairs to itself.

The reasoning goes that without using IF as a tool, even if we are eating in a way that continues ketosis through the day as well as overnight (which you of course are happily settled into now, having followed the shifts in part one of this book!) we aren't stimulating as much healing as we could.

Given that that muscle growth is vital to a healthy metabolism, the body will always prioritise healing and building muscle, bones, organs and skin over burning off excess fat stores. This can lead to unneeded scale frustration, as the pointless numbers aren't moving downwards.

However, if you know this fact, and especially if you have a past history of many nutrient barren low-fat diets, you can expect a "scale stall", relax and enjoy the benefits of a shrinking body instead.

One more body function of note is the interaction between Human Growth Hormone (HGH) and Insulin-like Growth Factor 1 (IGF-1) – IGF-1, as the name suggests, mimics the action of Insulin on cells and it is important for childhood cell growth.

However, lots of it running about in our bloodstream as adults causes accelerated cell aging as well as having been implicated as encouraging cancer cells to multiply.

Fasting increases human growth hormone (HGH) secretion[69] and decreases IGF-1 secretion. For proper growth, even as we grow older, we need alternating periods between HGH and IGF-1 being dominant, which IF gives us in a very efficient and pretty painless way.

IF also increases Brain Derived Neurotrophic Factor (BDNF) - "growth hormone for the brain" – and having a nice large amount of BDNF running around our brain helps it to grow in all ways, it encourages new neurons to grow, it encouraged neuroplasticity, which is our ability to learn new things as well as enhancing synaptic plasticity.

So, along with the controlling factor that IF has on Insulin, which promotes the brain using ketones rather than glucose, it also enhances the way that the glymphatic system operates. This system was only discovered in 2012, and it is the brain's overnight rubbish removal system.

---

[69] https://www.marksdailyapple.com/health-benefits-of-intermittent-fasting/

Encouraging the brain to work on ketones improves the function of our mitochondria as we sleep, turbo charging the whole of the glymphatic system.

High levels of BDNF, low levels of Insulin and excellent sleep habits have been shown to reduce the risk of Alzheimer's disease. IF is excellent for brain health as well as body health.

As you can see, by working gently to extend the fasted window by even a couple of hours, but ideally to around 16 hours per day, as well as feeding ourselves nutrient dense food within the eating window, we do many of good things for our body.

Also remember that the window is not one of caloric restriction, it's instead a time restriction. Eating enough fat to not get ravenously hungry during the fasting window is very important to overall health and happiness. You will almost certainly find that as your body settles into the rhythm of IF that you naturally begin to consume less food overall, but initially don't worry about quantity at all.

Also worth remembering, the autophagy process stops as soon as we chew something that stimulates even the tiniest bit of Insulin. This is why some people recommend that if you are hungry towards the end of the fasting window that drinking a small amount of fat, such as the butter and MCT oil in a "bulletproof coffee" (recipe in the printables supplement), a tsp of coconut oil melted and taken as a shot or a slug of double cream is enough to tide you over.

The reasoning behind this fat "not breaking the fasted state" is that pure fat doesn't stimulate Insulin. Your body sees both consumed fats and liberated body fats floating around the bloodstream as fodder for the Krebs cycle. And by drinking rather than eating this fat, you are not chewing and so not stimulating Insulin that way either.

There are other suggestions, such as a pinch of salt on the tongue followed by water, or a shot of apple cider vinegar with the mother[70] mixed into 500ml of water and sipped that also seem to curb hunger pangs and get us to the start of the eating window.

If you do fancy a bash at IF, do more research than I can give you in this small section[71]. As with all things low carb, your own research is gold.

Note that choosing to fast is not the same as starvation.

I've covered already what the body sees as starvation, the prolonged absence of all food, leading to the exhaustion of its fat reserves, and also what constitutes a semi-starvation diet.

---

[70]https://www.hollandandbarrett.com/the-health-hub/5-benefits-of-apple-cider-vinegar-with-the-mother/

[71]https://www.youtube.com/playlist?list=PL48jnTudSMf_7Ouf84s32g42Wx_DOwZBV

Such a diet was given to the participants of the Minnesota Starvation study[72] and the study found that it ramps down metabolism and preserves fat storage as long as possible in order to preserve life.

The diet given in the study was designed to emulate the foods that were expected to typify the diets of people in Europe during the latter stages world war II: , around 1500 Calories (depending on the subject, some men received as little as 1000 Calories) of mostly nutrient barren carbohydrate foods such as potatoes, swede, turnips, bread and pasta with very little fat or protein.

Does this maybe sound similar to other diets of your past at all?

As the diet fed in the study was almost exclusively carbohydrate, it kept Insulin elevated, and so it prevented body fat burning via ketosis and stopped the healing effects of autophagy from kicking in as well as not giving the hormone levelling effect of Leptin signalling.

The participants of the study complained of being cold all the time, were not at all interested in sex, exercise or socialising and were constantly hungry and totally food obsessed. They lost muscle mass, stamina and bone density.

---

[72]https://en.wikipedia.org/wiki/Minnesota_Starvation_Experiment

However, most people that use IF in conjunction with a low carb way of life find that their energy increases even more than with a more standard low carb eating pattern, they are rarely hungry once their body has a pattern it likes established and that they are willing and wanting to engage is all forms of socialisation and exercise.

People remark that others tell them that they "look younger", as the body is not wasting itself away and IF also has a powerful effect on the skin, causing it to tauten and "shrink back" in sync with the ditching of excess body fat.

So, if you do fancy having a bash at IF, how does it work? As I mentioned earlier, start gradually extending your fasting window, the bulk of which will be overnight.

Some people find that they want to eat more in the morning and so having an eating window that lasts until mid-afternoon works well for them, others find that not breaking their fast with brunch around noon and then having an eating window until around 8pm suits their lives better.

This having an elongated fast period every day is known as the 16:8 pattern – a 16-hour fasting window and an 8-hour eating window. You could go from 14:10 up to 20:4, it's whatever suits you and your life and body.

Pay attention to what your body is telling you – if you try and push a fasted window too hard, your body will respond and will demand you eat, and if you are not prepared, you may well find yourself going towards the non-optimal.

Others have five days in the week of "normal" eating, and then for 2 days, either together or separately, only eating 500-600 Calories of food. This 5:2 pattern appears to be less successful in terms of actually being able to sustain this way of eating over the long term, simply because unless you are willing to eat mostly fat to sustain yourself on your fast days, this will potentially be just enough food to lift the body out of overnight ketosis.

Whist a low carbohydrate way of doing 5:2 is sensible and not at all arduous, as bulletproof coffee, cream cheese, macadamia nuts and other high fat foods on fasting days would be an easy way of living, having read the books that suggest this method, they seem to instead offer a "low calorie, low fat, high carb" menu for both the "normal" and fasting days.

In my opinion, this is going to leave the person using the method of 5:2 as described with gut-gnawing hunger day-in-day-out, which is totally unsustainable long term.

Some people find that they naturally fall into fasting for one day a week, consuming mostly water with maybe a little drinkable fat if they get a hunger pang. The Pioppi protocol as promoted by UK cardiologist Dr Aseem Malhotra actively promotes doing this.

There is also nothing to stop you doing a prolonged water fast – stop eating and drink water only for at least 3 but preferably at least 5 days. As ketosis deepens appetite naturally declines, and the programmed "Ghrelin waves" that happen at what our bodies have learned are "meal times" lessen and eventually diminish after 72 hours for most people.

Some people that do water fasting aim to eat again when their body tells them they are hungry, which is usually around 10-12 days in this prolonged fasted state. [73]

As metabolism increases in a fasted state, don't be afraid to do some exercise if you feel the need; a good walk, some yoga or a round of resistance work. Let your body tell you what it wants to do, do move but don't push so hard that your body demands some energy input!

The bottom line is that if you are going to incorporate IF into your regimen, find out what suits you, and even if IF suits your body at all... some people love it, others find that it's simply not for them. As I said, it's not at all obligatory to use IF along with a low carb way of eating, however, even extending your overnight fasting window by a couple of hours will boost autophagy and it can be useful in terms of overall heath as well as specifically boosting brain health.

---

[73] https://youtu.be/APZCfmgzoS0

Our brains on sugar

Talking of our brains... The brain is our most energy demanding organ, its mass only constitutes ~2% of the entire body weight, however, it demands and consumes around 20% of our body's total energy output[74]

Insulin is extremely efficient at its job and because of this, when Insulin is wandering about mob-handed, glucose levels can drop to a point where our brain senses there is not enough glucose hanging around it to make energy from, as well as not hearing Leptin telling it that our fat cells are full and that we don't need to eat more because there is plenty of energy to liberate if only it wanted to do so.

When our bodies are running in a high carbohydrate situation, our brain is extremely demanding for glucose. As we've discussed, as we carry on eating carbs over time, the Insulin surge followed by blood glucose crash, causes the brain to demand more glucose, which then causes another Insulin surge and glucose crash.

Having our blood sugar surge and crash all the time is not at all healthy or even how evolution designed us to be.

---

[74] Drubach, Daniel. The Brain Explained. New Jersey: Prentice-Hall, 2000. Pg 161
https://books.google.co.uk/books?id=hcVqAAAAMAAJ
And
"The fat-fueled brain: unnatural or advantageous?"
https://blogs.scientificamerican.com/mind-guest-blog/the-fat-fueled-brain-unnatural-or-advantageous/

As we evolved, our brains ran mostly on ketones, not on glucose – using the same mechanisms we are exploiting when eating a low carbohydrate diet.

One of the things that happens to our body and brain when lots of glucose is running about is increased incidence of plaques – in our arteries, plaques are made from LDL but in the brain, they are abnormal clusters of chemically "sticky" proteins called beta-amyloid.

It's these beta-amyloid plaques that lead to Alzheimer's, and so some researchers have started to call it "Type III diabetes,"[75] as they've pinpointed resistance to Insulin and Insulin-like growth factor as being a key part of the progression of Alzheimer's disease. [76]

And talking of diabetes...

---

[75]https://www.biosciencetechnology.com/article/2015/05/diabetes-sugars-and-alzheimers-brain-plaques-potentially-linked
https://www.diabetes.co.uk/type3-diabetes.html and https://insulinresistance.org/index.php/jir/article/view/15/32 as notable articles - there is plenty to read on this subject!

[76] Rhode Island Hospital Study Finds Link Between Brain Insulin Resistance and Neuronal Stress in Worsening Alzheimer's Disease
Neurosciences Institute, Research, RIH. June 26, 2012
http://www.rhodeislandhospital.org/wtn/Page.asp?PageID=WTN000249

Diabetes

At its heart, Diabetes Mellitus, to give it its full medical name is a disease of carbohydrate intolerance.

Diabetes is an old disease. During the second century CE Aretaeus of Cappadocia wrote a clinical description any doctor, nurse or patient today would readily recognise for type I diabetes:

'Diabetes ... is a melting down of the flesh and limbs into urine. The patients never stop making water and the flow is incessant, like the opening of aqueducts. Life is short, unpleasant and painful. The patients' thirst is unquenchable, their drinking is excessive ... and within a short time they expire." 77

He went on to write that *'The disease appears to have got its name from the Greek for siphon."* as the disease is characterised by diuresis or excessive peeing; the words 'diuresis' and 'diuretic' derive from the Greek words for 'through' and 'urine'.

———————————

[77] Adapted from Laios et al. (2012), 'Arataeus of Cappadocia and the first description of diabetes', Hormones 11: 109-13.

Sushruta, the Father of Indian Surgery, described two types of diabetes mellitus in his *Sushruta Samhita*, a medical text written in the fifth century CE:

> '*Sweet is the urine … This disease may be ascribed to two causes, the congenital and that attributable to an injudicious diet … The former type is associated with emaciation, the latter with obesity and an inclination for lounging in bed or on cushions.*'[78]

Following the fall of the Roman Empire and the descent of Europe into the Dark Ages, where it wasn't really at all fashionable to write stuff down as they were too busy simply surviving complex political failures and successive waves of invaders from all sides, there is no real evidence of further advances on Aretaeus's or Sushruta's clinical descriptions of diabetes until the seventeenth century, when Dr Thomas Willis (1621-75) of Oxford started the process of classifying diabetes into two major categories, diabetes insipidus and diabetes mellitus.

The obvious distinction he made was that in mellitus the urine is sweet (because it's full of glucose; 'mellitus' coming from the Greek *meli* for 'honey') whereas in insipidus is, well, insipid!

In the past the differential diagnosis was made by doctors tasting the urine, a task generally delegated to the most junior member of the team. Thankfully now, we have urinalysis sticks!

---

[78] Quoted in Richard Dods (2013), Understanding Diabetes: A Biochemical Perspective, John Wiley, New Jersey, pp. 27-8.

Diabetes insipidus is a very rare disorder caused by problems with a hormone called Vasopressin (AVP) (also called antidiuretic hormone (ADH)) and has no link to diabetes mellitus at all.

Because the disease involves a diuresis, or excess, of urine, diabetes insipidus retains the name given to it back in the 17th century. However, it's fundamentally different from diabetes mellitus, so we don't need to go into it any further.

There are two major types of diabetes mellitus, the thankfully rare type I and the increasingly common type II. Regardless of differing causes, their shared characteristic of high levels of blood glucose means that they also share certain complications as persistently elevated blood glucose levels gradually destroy the eyes, kidneys, nerves and small blood vessels over time.

Type I diabetes is an auto-immune disease; for reasons unknown to science at this time, the body attacks itself and totally kills off the beta-cells in the islets of Langerhans, located in the pancreas.

The beta-cells make Insulin, and so type I is a disease of total Insulin absence, which allows blood glucose levels to soar out of control, until the kidneys step in and start continually dumping glucose into the urine, causing intense thirst.

As Insulin also guides glucose into the cells so that ATP can be easily made, the body cannot use any of the ample glucose running around. So, the body starts breaking down muscle protein to make more glucose for energy, which of course without Insulin, it also also cannot use.

Also, because Insulin is not around to keep fat locked up in the fat cells, they empty out, liberating fatty acids into the blood stream for the mitochondria to pick and use for energy.

This is what leads to the dramatic reduction in both lean and fatty body mass seen in (usually) children that develop type I diabetes.

The final nail in the coffin however is that fatty acids in the blood in combination with high levels of glucose turn the blood acidic – this is known as diabetic ketoacidosis[79] and will cause coma and swift death if left unresolved.

Until 1921, when Sir Frederick Grant Banting KBE MC FRS FRSC discovered and isolated Insulin from pancreatic cells and then swiftly moved in 1922 to treat the first human type I patient[80], type I diabetes was classified as a swift moving terminal illness. Banting's work has given an extended life span to people with type I diabetes worldwide.

Type II happens when the Insulin resistance caused by constantly eating too much carbohydrate becomes so great that blood glucose remains at a high level because

---

[79] https://en.wikipedia.org/wiki/Diabetic_ketoacidosis

[80] https://web.archive.org/web/20180809191513/https://www.nobelprize.org/educational/medicine/insulin/discovery-insulin.html

even Insulin's action "mob-handed" is no longer enough to unlock the cells to let in glucose consistently and so blood glucose levels remain constantly elevated and health starts to deteriorate.

If blood glucose is left totally uncontrolled, the pancreas eventually fills with fat, the beta cells "burn out" and then stop producing Insulin altogether.

Then raging thirst and increased hunger develops, as well as blurry vision, fatigue and a sudden unexpected reduction in both lean and fatty body mass, identical to what is seen in a type I diabetic patient, but for a different reason.

Caught early enough and treated correctly with a low carbohydrate diet, the pancreatic fat can be removed and given time and rest, the beta-cells of many patients can recover their function.

However, current treatment guidelines (medicate around the problems) prevent the beta-cells from resting and so doom a type II patient to a life of drugs and bad blood glucose control leading to inevitable health complications.

As Sushruta observed, type II tends to develop in people "who are obese and physically inactive" and once diagnosed in our current system, the person starts a long grind into "sickness management" with first medication to reduce blood glucose levels and then as the disease progresses, Insulin injections to control blood glucose.

All this rather than simply telling patients to stop eating the food that is giving the issues, sugar and starchy carbohydrates. Which until the 70's was exactly what patients with diabetes were told!

As diabetes is a firm indicator of CHD risk, and with the vilification of fats in the 70's and 80's, treatment shifted away from carbohydrate restriction and toward the opinion that the "standard diet being suitable for diabetics" with blood glucose control being achieved more via drugs rather than diet.

The current advice is that people with diabetes are told to lower their fat content and regulate their caloric intake over all, to attempt to prevent obesity. Which as we know, is counter to the way that our endocrine system works.

Thankfully, the tide is now turning. Although many CCG's and the Diabetes UK website,[81] (the main diabetes charity in the UK) still recommend a high carbohydrate diet based around conventional "healthy eating" there is an up-swell of sense from some CCGs, as well as GPs and Diabetic nurses acting independently who are now going against the NHS guidelines and recommending a low carbohydrate diet as the first line of diabetes treatment.

There are also an increasing number of people fed up with being sick with diabetes taking their own treatment in hand. The Diabeties.co.uk website, which is a

---

[81]https://www.diabetes.org.uk/Guide-to-diabetes/Enjoy-food/Eating-with-diabetes/What-is-a-healthy-balanced-diet

community website for people with diabetes, has an article critiquing the NHS position[82] and has launched a website specifically focused on treatment of Type II diabetes via a Low Carb diet
https://www.lowcarbprogram.com/

I personally always recommend that people coming to low carb with diabetes look up Dr Bernstein, a type I diabetic born in 1934.

His life story is fascinating[83] and all about how in 1969, after his doctor told him "it's impossible to normalize human blood sugars", he used his engineer brain to work the problem.

He asked his MD wife to buy him a $650 blood glucose testing machine meant for hospital use only and figured out how to perfectly balance his Insulin and control his blood glucose via experimentation on himself. He then went and qualified as an MD, so that he could get his work recognised and help other people with diabetes.

His books are what I consider to be the gold standard in diabetes care.

I prefer "Dr Bernstein's Diabetes diet" to "Dr Bernstein's Diabetes solution" as it is an easier read, aimed at lay

---

[82]https://www.diabetes.co.uk/diet/low-carb-diets-and-nhs-advice.html

[83]http://www.diabetes-book.com/bernstein-life-with-diabetes/

people, whereas "Diabetes solution" feels firmly pitched more at the medical community.

However, I think that both books are invaluable and work well as a pair, as Dr B references the more complex "Diabetes Solution" throughout "Diabetes Diet" https://amzn.to/2uwlGw4 [84]

Dr B's work is also the reason why we now have hand-held glucometers for easy patient self-management. If you don't own one and have diabetes, I urge you to do some research into the best machine for you and purchase one. You are only issued one and supplies routinely by the NHS if you have type I diabetes or if your type II becomes type I due to pancreatic burn-out.

A fantastic concept that uses the glucometer to best effect is "The Law of Small Numbers" – Doing experiments on yourself to discover how you react to carbohydrate and protein food, and charting what's going on over a 24 hr period over several weeks so that you can work how and what keeps your blood glucose within a 5-point plus or minus variation at all times.

---

[84] Something to remember is that blood glucose readings in America are measured in different units to nigh on the entire rest of the world! They use mg/dL whereas we use mmol/L.
Use this handy converter as required - https://www.diabetes.co.uk/blood-sugar-converter.html - and don't let that put you off reading or doing your own research on the internet.

I mention protein here because of gluconeogenesis – if you aren't expecting it, protein can throw your numbers out, so someone with diabetes has to aim for consistency in both carb and protein at each meal, and enough fat to ensure that you have no need to snack, so that your blood glucose numbers are not thrown off.

Another thing to note when living with diabetes is also related to gluconeogenesis - the dawn phenomenon. I mentioned it earlier in the section on Cortisol, and this phenomenon is a major factor for people with diabetes to consider in their overall health regimen.

The dawn phenomenon peaks blood glucose because Cortisol is breaking down protein to give a glucose boost to get the body moving at the start of the day. This means that your blood glucose will rise in the first few hours of your day after waking.

This means that for someone with diabetes, breakfast will ideally be much lower in carbohydrate than the other two meals of the day. Dr B suggests starting your experiments with 30g of carbs a day, spilt 6g:12g:12g.

You may also find that you can do without breakfast at all, and intermittent fasting with two equally sized meals a day could sit well with your diabetes management.

If you are taking medication for your diabetes, simply put, you are going to find you need less of it. Medication such as Gliclazide, which forces the pancreas to pump out more Insulin and Metformin, an Insulin sensitizer given to overcome cell Insulin resistance are prescribed to overcome the effects of a standard high carb diet on a diabetic body.

Note that I'm not a Doctor or in any way medically qualified. I talk a good talk because I've done extensive research in how the body works. However, you **must** work with your doctor to establish your new baseline of needed medication. I am not offering you medical advice, instead I am showing you potential avenues of explorations that you can take with your doctor.

You may find them resistant to your choice, after all, you are going against the current NHS guidelines and you may not live in an enlightened NHS trust.

The other reason you may meet resistance is simply that some GPs don't like their patients taking control of their own health. Not every doctor is open to that, or even to new ideas.

I've also heard people say that their doctors and diabetes clinics tell them "we can't condone what you are doing, but your numbers are fantastic, keep doing what you are doing!" As I've mentioned, the tide is slowly turning, and prominent doctors within the NHS are now getting on board with a low carb treatment path for diabetes. Right now, it bodes well for the future health of the nation.

In my life, and in this book, you will have seen that I'm laid back when it comes to not really counting anything and simply eating to hunger within the OSN scale via making mostly optimal choices.

However, if you have diabetes, life is necessarily one of stringent food discipline if health and vitality are to be preserved. The discipline can reverse complications as much as is possible for the body to heal as well as preventing the common diabetic complications from happening if implemented early enough.

It's not unknown for type II diabetes to totally vanish with a well thought out low carb regimen, as removing the main cause of the disease (refined carbohydrate) allows the pancreas to have a rest and recharge its Insulin making abilities whilst allowing the body's Insulin sensitivity to fall back to more natural levels.

And whilst I'm not promising that will happen for you, the healing that you will see through removing the substance that is causing your disease will improve your life overall.

The gut microbiome

I could have called this section "the case for not being afraid to eat your vegetables." Why? Because the fibre and phytonutrients we gain from eating a diverse selection of vegetables and other whole food are in my view essential for a healthy and diverse collection of bacteria in our guts.[85] And one of the best ways to maintain the health of our gut microbiome is by eating a diverse non-processed food diet with a good selection of colourful vegetables.

I've been living a low carb life and hosting low carb mailing lists and Facebook groups for the last 18 years, and I've seen a great deal of people that follow the "stay under 20g of Carbohydrate a day" dictum that, as far as I can tell, Dr Atkins' gifted the world back in 1972 and so many authors have picked up on and used ever after.

I look at this dictum and see it as woefully detrimental for a few reasons, one of the most important being in terms of the food that it forces people to remove from their diets.

One of the reasons that I feel that this restrictive level of carbs could be harmful is by discouraging regular consumption of the slightly starchier colourful vegetables – the one's that I view as suboptimal.

Doctors such as Dr David Perlmutter and Dr Michael Mosely argue that the main reason for us as humans to

---

[85] https://youtu.be/1sISguPDlhY

eat vegetative fibre is not to feed ourselves, but to feed our gut microbiome. There is also good evidence that we have evolved to live symbiotically with our gut bacteria, as a major component of breast milk is "Human milk oligosaccharides" (HMO), a family of structurally diverse unconjugated glycans that are found in and unique to human breast milk.

They function as a prebiotic for "our first microbiome,"-the Bifidobacteria longum biovar infantis[86] bacteria that are found in breast milk and the birth canal. HMO feeds the bacteria that the baby swallows at birth and during feeding and helping to encourage the baby's gut to develop its own microbiome.

A healthy and diverse gut microbiome is one of the keys to our long-term health, as one of the roles of the microbiome is to help us digest our food. As I mentioned earlier, differences in microbiome mean that if you feed the same plateful of food to a room full of people, they will all extract differing amounts of nutrients and energy from it. On top of this, the microbes in our microbiome could also influence our chances of becoming obese or staying slender.

How do we know this? Very recently, a medical process called "faecal microbiota transplant" has been developed, which is where poo from a screened healthy donor is "reseeded" into a patient who is suffering from clostridium difficile infection (CDI) or whose own gut microbiome has totally died off for whatever reason.

---

[86] https://en.wikipedia.org/wiki/Bifidobacterium_longum

However, there have been cases where the person receiving the faecal donation can become the shape of their donor[87] [88]!

Whilst the science around this is still very much being investigated, there is a pointer in the data to the quality of our gut microbiome being linked to the storage of body fat, either in a positive or negative way.

However, let's take a step back though and ask why the composition of our gut microbiome is so important.

When we talk about "gut feeling" we are reflecting the truth that our entire digestive tract is lined with neurons, around 100 million of them, and the neurons in our gut are closely tied into our intuitive process, when we "just know" if something is right or wrong. When you compare this to the fact that the brain itself contains around 100 billion neurons, you can see that the enteric system, or "second brain" that sits in your gut is not at all insignificant in the grand scheme of things.

The primary input that our gut neurons receive about the world is derived from food. The enteric system has open two-way communication with the brain via the vagus nerve, which is the main nerve pathway of the parasympathetic nervous system[89].

---

[87] https://www.newscientist.com/article/mg22530083-600-not-just-obesity-faecal-transplants-weird-effects/

[88] https://www.livescience.com/59063-fecal-transplants-weight-changes.html

[89] https://en.wikipedia.org/wiki/Vagus_nerve

The communication channel is also be used by our microbiome[90], and the microbes also produce a range of hormone-like chemicals and neurotransmitters that reach the brain via the bloodstream. These manipulate us into eating what they need to survive and reward us when we do as they want.

For example, the microbes in your gut produce lots of dopamine as a reward when we feed them correctly. They also produce chemicals that control mood, such as serotonin and GABA (a neurotransmitter than acts in a similar way to diazepam). They even make chemicals that are almost identical to Leptin and Ghrelin!

There is also increasing and interesting research on how our gut microbiome influences and affects the structure of our brain and its myelinisation.[91] Dr Aktipis, from the Arizona State University Department of Psychology says, "Microbes have the capacity to manipulate behaviour and mood through altering the neural signals in the vagus nerve, changing taste receptors, producing toxins to make us feel bad and releasing chemical rewards to make us feel good,"

She collaborated on a major review of the scientific literature in 2014, which asked the question: 'Is eating behaviour manipulated by the gastrointestinal microbiota?'

---

[90]https://www.ncbi.nlm.nih.gov/pmc/articles/PMC4367 209/

[91]https://www.theguardian.com/science/neurophilosoph y/2016/apr/05/gut-bacteria-brain-myelin

The answer was a resounding 'yes'. They put together a convincing case that microbes not only influence how much we eat but what we eat.[92][93]

When the gut microbiome is balanced between a wide variety of our most helpful microbes, the ones that consume fats as well as the ones that consume sugars. we stay healthy. Because our microbiome is happy, we are also happy and tend to have a lot of energy.

However, we generally suffer a host of health issues, such as weight gain, diabetes, brain fog, and maybe even cancer when the microbiome has been thrown out by a junk-food diet. The microbes that love junk food and sugar very much encourage us to eat more of the food they need to thrive, so that they can become the dominant culture in our digestive tracts, which then throws the whole body out of whack!

Yet another reason why becoming fat is probably not your fault, your gut microbiome may well have been influencing you to eat more crap!

However, the average lifespan of a microbiome microbe is around 20 minutes, so we have the opportunity every

---

[92] "Is eating behavior manipulated by the gastrointestinal microbiota?" Evolutionary pressures and potential mechanisms. BioEssays, 2014

[93]

https://www.theguardian.com/lifeandstyle/2017/nov/06/micromicrobiome-gut-health-digestive-system-genes-happiness time we eat to work towards changing the population of the gut microbiome.

As well as eating the colourful and prebiotic vegetables, such as garlic, asparagus, radishes, leeks, Jerusalem artichokes, and carrots, eating prebiotic fermented food, such as yoghurt, kefir, kimchee, sauerkraut, tempeh and kombucha is also a good thing for our microbiome diversity.

Turmeric has also been shown to have a positive effect on the microbiome, as well as an anti-inflammatory effect on the gut wall itself. It also boosts bile production and the secretion of protective stomach mucus[94].

Omega-3 fatty acids such as DHA also boost biome diversity, so adding oily fish to your diet a few times a week is also up there, especially if you are an older woman.[95]

Finally, getting out in the fresh air, or even opening a window as well as gardening and getting a bit grubby whilst out and about in nature can massively drive diversity in the microbiome.

Taking a high-quality probiotic can also be useful, especially if you know that courses of antibiotics have depleted your microbiome.

---

[94]https://www.globalhealingcenter.com/natural-health/can-turmeric-support-gut-health/

[95]https://www.medicalnewstoday.com/articles/319375.php

If you do this, remember to keep the bottle in the fridge, and don't take the capsule with a hot beverage! Probiotics are living microbes, and heat is death to them, turning an expensive product into a waste of cash.

A high-quality probiotic is measured in "colony forming units" (CFUs) and the higher this number the better! Look for

- ❖ a CFU of between 5-10 billion, in a daily capsule
- ❖ an "enteric" capsule that can survive transit through stomach acid,
- ❖ a product that contains more than one strain of microbe
- ❖ a product that includes species of Lactobacillus and Bifidobacterium.
    - ❖ Lactobacillus acidophilus and Lactobacillus plantarum reside in the small intestine and the upper GI tract among your immune cells.
    - ❖ Bifidobacterium lactis, Bifidobacterium longum, and Bifidobacterium bifidum reside in the large intestine and lower bowel.

Having a healthy gut microbiome also promotes regular bowel functions, which takes me nicely into talking about poo itself.

Constipation

Constipation is not the lack of stool per se, it is the consistency of the stool itself. Less need to poo isn't constipation.

Us brits come up with all the cool ideas about poo! One of these is the "Bristol Stool Scale[96]", detailing seven degrees of stool consistency, from one: "separate hard lumps" through to seven: "liquid with no solid pieces."

Three and four are the "desirable consistency" for human poo, a three being "a sausage shape with crack in the surface" and four being a "smooth and soft sausage or snake-like stool"

Due to the lack of rubbish that the body cannot use in your diet now, you are almost certainly going to find your stool is a little smaller, and the bowel moves less frequently than before. For some people, having a more frequent movement than before happens initially as gut bacteria that feed on sugars die off, and the intestines work to remove it. All this is natural and to be expected.

You may also find your movements a touch harder, dipping down into a 2 on the scale if you aren't eating enough vegetables, fat or drinking enough water.

Fat also encourages peristalsis, the waves of muscle that move food through the gut, which is another reason why

———————————————————————

[96] https://en.wikipedia.org/wiki/Bristol_stool_scale

eating a fatty breakfast is good, as it encourages a morning movement.

How much water the solid matter picks up in transit influences the hardness of our stool, and electrolytes have an influence as they keep the body's water balance correct.

Eating too little sodium leads to water being pulled out of the body via the kidney's, which means that there is not enough in the bowel to soften the stool in transit.

So, the best cures for low carb connected constipation are:

- ❖ eating more greens and vegetable fibre
  - o to provide bulk and food for the gut microbiome
- ❖ eating more fat
  - o to encourage peristalsis
- ❖ drinking more water
  - o to provide water to soften the stool
- ❖ balancing your electrolytes (https://amzn.to/2q33XIf)
  - o so that water stays in your bowel where you need it
- ❖ taking 400mg of Magnesium Citrate or 35-40ml of Milk of Magnesia before bed
- ❖ having an Epsom salt (Magnesium Sulphate) bath before bed.
  - o Both relax the gut, encourage peristalsis and work to soften stool.

❖ moving more during your day

○ Moving around helps the bowel to move itself, and sitting for long periods is not a good idea if you want a softer stool

And that final point moves me squarely onto the interesting subject of exercise.

Exercise

Otherwise known as the other arm of "eat less, move more and all your troubles melt away…"

Whilst I'm 100% in favour of exercise, as it is excellent for overall health as well as a serious mood elevator, it's absolutely useless as a "weight loss tool." I've had serious disagreements with people on Facebook over this point.

It's a fact that if you have a biscuit, no amount of exercise will ever "run off the calories" or negate the hormonal effects that a carb based non-optimal choice has on the body.

As we know, it's not about calories, it's about what the food you eat does to our hormones. Exercise does not reduce Insulin, the only thing that does do that is not eating carbohydrates! It does however reduce any Cortisol release stimulated by stress, making it our best tool to actively reduce the physiological stress factors.

As a species, we evolved to move and lift things, build all manner of structures, walk and run places, climb trees and hills and jump over rocky terrain. In modern life though, we spend way too much time sitting on our bums and not doing any of these things; this is such a shame, as exercise also improves skeletal muscle Insulin sensitivity, and makes the Krebs cycle run faster, giving us even more energy at our disposal.

So, having established that exercise is a generally good thing, doing as much as you feel is right for you is also a good thing. Which, especially if you have a significant amount of fat to drop right now can be no exercise. One of the results of an imbalanced metabolism where the body's hormones are rigged towards storage rather than expenditure is that there isn't excess energy available to exercise.

What many people find as their hormone systems normalise with eating a healthy low carbohydrate diet is that they spontaneously get the urge to move around more. They wonder what on earth is up, where is all this energy coming from? Well, it's coming out of your fat cells! The body is finally able to mobilise and access all that stored energy it's been lugging about and it starts spending it with joy!

So, what's my very subjective opinion on exercise in terms of body composition and health? Well, I personally love yoga. It's a good combination of resistance and cardio.

After all, we need both in the right proportions for body balance. Anabolic (muscle building) resistance work, such as lugging the shopping back from the shops, gardening or any other pursuit that moves heavy things around slowly, builds our muscles which increases energy metabolism over the long term. This is because the muscle mitochondria is the main place the Krebs cycles runs, and so our body makes ATP mostly in our muscles.

There is also a need for a touch of cardio, for instance a good brisk walk of around 20 mins everyday, as this promotes stamina as well as BDNF production.

Which I know goes against the classic advice of "cardio, cardio, cardio!!!" – I am strongly against extended cardio sessions because of its catabolic effects. Put simply, catabolic exercise means muscle breakdown, which is not what anyone wants out of a workout.

We are taught that extended cardio sessions will "make the fat melt off because it burns calories", but it is simply not the case. You can't use energy if you have no muscles to create ATP!

It's very beneficial for women to focus more in resistance work. Strong muscles equal strong bones. And strong bones are a preventative against osteoporosis when we start perimenopause, as the decrease in Oestrogen also has an effect on bone density.

Although resistance work for both sexes is important, the male body has more muscle density to start with and women are not encouraged to be strong by society. As I spoke about earlier, a woman with a healthy musculature is seen as rather freakish and undesirable by society. So much so that the muscles on more athletic woman are routinely smoothed out and erased by the use of Photoshop[97].

---

[97]https://www.shape.com/celebrities/celebrity-photos/12-celebs-airbrushed-look-bigger-and-less-muscular and https://youtu.be/g6eRzOMbOf8

However, having a healthy musculature, and I'm not talking muscle bulging out everywhere, slows aging and helps to prevent "frailty issues" as we age, such as major injury from slips, trips and falls.

Regular resistance work decreases blood pressure, which is increasingly important as we age. It also increases production of all myokines which, amongst other things improve glucose uptake in our muscles, increases lipolysis in our fat cells and reduces cancer risk factors. BDNF is also a myokine, and resistance increases circulating BDNF as well.[98]

As you can tell, I do think that exercising the heart to build stamina is important, but I'm more strongly in favour of doing regular resistance work! I'm also in favour of doing as much exercise as you are able to do, without putting pressure on yourself to go nuts with it because you feel you have to do it.

[98]https://www.ncbi.nlm.nih.gov/pmc/articles/PMC4657151/

The stall – why they have to happen for your health

Firstly, let's define what a stall is - A stall is when there is no change to both body weight and body measurements for four weeks or more.

Most people have been trained that they make progress only when the scale number is dropping, and that it should drop consistently and constantly. So, if the scale has not moved for a few days to a week, they will begin to mix things up when there is no need to do so.

For your health, stalls must happen, they are a simple fact of life. When we choose to purposefully start burning away our fat stores, and especially if we try to force the body to go faster, the body has no way of knowing that we have chosen to reduce our size.

Our mind knows we've made a change and that we want to sustain it over time, whereas our body lives in the now, and assesses the situation moment to moment. It wants to maintain homeostasis – the current status quo - to ensure we stay alive. When it sees is a change, it tries to figure out what is happening and attempts to maintain homeostasis.

"Woah, what's happening right now???" it says to itself, "There is some serious fat store depletion going on, something must be wrong! Hold stations everyone, we need to figure out what's happening!"

When the scale is not moving, two mechanisms are at play. They can happen either separately or together.

1. The body resists change, and its protective mechanisms are in full effect. Neither the scale nor the tape measure show moment.
2. The body is gaining muscle mass and burning fat at an equal rate. Measurements reduce but the scale reflects "no change".

The first mechanism causes a period of conservation, the body ramps down various mechanisms. This is so that you can stay alive as long as possible, given the current conditions. In a low calorie/low fat situation, where muscle is also being consumed due to calorie and protein deficit, this actively and permanently slows the metabolism.

However, in the case of low carb eating, where nutrient dense food is not restricted and the body is not consuming its own muscle mass, all that is needed is to simply keeping doing what you are doing. This lets the body know that energy and body building blocks - protein and dietary fat - are plentiful. What is happening is the new normal, there is no emergency. And that it doesn't need to hoard the stores.

The body not realising there is a new normal in some people can take months. Especially if there is a great deal of muscle and bone depletion damage to heal caused by previous cycles of low fat, low protein eating.

Yes, this is a hard thing to hear. But remember that every mouthful of nutritionally dense food is improving your body and your health.

The second reason only causes the scale to stop moving. In my opinion, the scale is the worst way of measuring progress. This is the main reason why I hate using the nonspecific word weight when what we want to drop is fat.

If the body has been previously damaged by cycles of muscle reducing low fat dieting, the body will prioritise rebuilding itself over getting generally slimmer. When given a proper amount of fat and protein, muscle gain/body repair happens. This means that whilst the body is happily burning away fat it is also adding muscle.

Yes, this gives a stall on the scale, but the body is becoming denser and more metabolically active. And that is a very fine thing indeed.

Where we have been trained to become obsessed with the scale number, we lose sight of the fact that our body is becoming healthier as well as shrinking. The diet industry has sold us on only caring about the number on the scale, which is very counterproductive for sanity.

Worth remembering, fat is a whopping 17% less dense than muscle. It literally takes up 17% more space than the same amount of muscle in your body. Take a look at the picture on the next page, and you will see exactly what I mean!

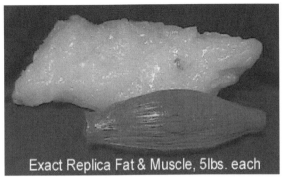

Exact Replica Fat & Muscle, 5lbs. each

Yes, stalls are very annoying, but you will be eating this way for the rest of your life, so why rush now? Your body's homoeostasis level needs time to "catch up and reset" with where you are and where you want to be going forward.

It took us all many years of non-healthy eating to get fat. Being impatient with the process of reversing the damage your previous diet caused is illogical, counterproductive for your mindset and in terms of your heath, not a good thing to do to your body.

Relax and enjoy the process of getting a lean and optimal body. After all, relaxing will lower your Cortisol levels and eating low carb is not exactly an arduous way of eating!

Also, LCHF will not let you drop under a healthy lean weight. Hence the "stubborn last7lbs" phenomenon - that last 7lbs is all wonderfully metabolically active muscle, & your body wants to keep it! Which leads me nicely on to...

The "Last 7 lbs is being stubborn" dilemma - this is why it really should not bother you!

One of the things that is most likely to discourage anyone slimming down is not reaching their (self-)assigned goal weight. Even with the luxury that is low-carb eating, not seeing those pesky "I'm at Goal!" digits showing on a set of scales can be annoying and disheartening.

Whilst I very much encourage people to go by what the tape measure says, most people are unfortunately still wedded to the scale number, and generally, people pick (or are assigned) a goal weight according to charts based on BMI[99]

BMI is a "population guide" and is known to be flawed at an individual level, as it takes no account at all of body composition. According to BMI, all Rugby players, body builders and other "strong" athletes with plenty of muscle mass but not much fat mass are ranked as "overweight" and "obese".

Because BMI is not at all reflective of body composition, most people that eat a healthy LCHF diet will never "lose the last 7lbs", and neither would they want to do so!

Those last 3Kg are metabolically active muscle which our bodies want to keep a hold on.

_____

[99] http://www.nhs.uk/Livewell/loseweight/Pages/height-weight-chart.aspx

This is where society does us no favours at all, as linguistically, it conflates the coverall term "weight" with our size and also our health.

This conflation of size with weight is shown wonderfully by Adrienne Osuna in her Instagram post in January 2017: https://www.instagram.com/p/BPacQ2lg3Us

When you look at the two pictures she took of herself side by side at 82.5Kg (182lb) vs 81.6Kg (180lb), your brain may well take a side step and tell you that she has to have dropped at least 7kgs! Because you have been trained to conflate size with weight. Breaking away from that training is one of the best things that you can do for your sanity.

As we know, muscle takes up 17% less space in the body than our fat does, so in terms of the scale, a person that has gained their slim and healthy body with low-carb eating usually weighs ~2-4Kg above the mid-range of where BMI says that we should be to be "ideal weight".

Remember, eating a healthy low-carb diet means that our bodies will not drop to an unhealthy body mass, at least, not without it protesting a massive amount at us as we impose too artificially strict restrictions on it!

Our bodies are slightly heavier but smaller & far more metabolically active than the bodies of people that have used "conventional wisdom" to starve their bodies of muscle as well as fat.

Let's state the obvious - male and female bodies have different physiologies

It's one of those things that the medical and scientific community tend to overlook, that physiologically, men and women aren't the same. Yes, our biology is mostly similar, but there are crucial differences in hormone levels that mean we are not the same.

It's a fact that men can drop their fat stores far faster than women - The male body is naturally more muscular, and so can drop fat more easily than the female body. The male physiology is also much less "lipophilic" than a women's physiology, women naturally carry more fat to make milk for babies and our boobs are mostly fatty tissue as well.

On the upside, female fat reserves are stored in far less injurious to health places usually - on the hips, thighs and boobs, and mostly subcutaneous (under the skin), where it isn't causing an issue, beyond the aesthetic and load bearing.

Men store their fat mostly viscerally (with and attached to the organs), which impinges on organ function and is a definite correlation to all the diseases of civilisation.

So, in my opinion, one of the worst things that a husband and wife team can do is "diet together to see who can lose the most / the fastest" - the man will always "win" that particular contest and this usually then makes the woman feel shitty about herself as she compares her body to his, and wonders why she is not getting the same result whilst doing the same thing as her husband.

So, whilst having a supportive partner is always a good thing, know that you are both on your own journeys. Remembering this will save lots of all round heartache.

Oh my gosh, my hair's falling out! What's that all about?

This is medically called "telogen effluvium." Hair growth has three phases, and telogen is the name for the hair follicles' resting state. The resting cycle of all the follicles is normally random, so that we don't lose lots of hair all at once.

However, after any "shock to the system" such as an extreme diet change, bereavement, divorce or accident, for some reason, the hair follicles all synchronise their telogen phase. This leads to seemingly sudden hair loss 3 months or so after the body shock event.

Don't worry about this, your hair won't all fall out and the follicle growth phases will sort themselves out. Your hair will easily grow back in a few months, and given the increase in protein and fats, usually becomes stronger and more lustrous than before.

Why I personally don't like the 20g limit of other "low carb diets"

Dr Atkins gave us the 20g limit in "Dr Atkins' Low Carb revolution" in 1972, written as "start here, and increase" guidance, but then people didn't increase because they wanted to "lose weight faster" – and it's been adopted by various low carb writers as "the golden number" where people need to be to get results.

Dr. Andreas Eenfeldt, the "Diet Doctor" is one of the most popular Low Carb writers at this time, and he is starting people off at 20g of carbs per day and leaving them there. I think, in terms of a healthy balanced life, that such a restrictive limit is a big disservice to human kind.

It's a disservice because most people don't need a "medical" level of ketosis - and applying treatments for sick people to a healthy population can be counter-productive. So, I personally feel that a "20g ketosis limit" is unhelpful to us for long term success.

I also think it better to start gradually and then move up or down from there, rather than do all in all at once and give the body a huge shock.

This is why I suggest back the introduction that once you have transitioned with the shifts, seeing how you go at around 50g and to tweak around, up or down as required.

The body adapts to what we give it, and I've seen hundreds of people, including myself, complain of long stalls and even fat gains if they eat even 5g over "their 20g" after around 8 months to a year or so.

As I mentioned in the gut biome section, having a 20g daily carbohydrate limit also cuts out the suboptimal vegetables that are higher on the carb scale but have massive nutrition power. Vegetables are always a good thing.

Yes, the human body can do very well on just "meat and leafy veg" - but not many people can sustain that level of restriction over a lifetime - even if they are not hungry from eating protein and fat "ad libitum".

We simply get bored and then seek variety - which can then cause issues. I know for me, that was one of my issues the first time around - but then, I was making a heck of a lot of non-optimal "junk food" choices as well! 18 years ago, Dove's gluten free lemon biscuits covered with clotted cream was my favourite in this category. The combo of fat and fast acting starchy carbs really is very non-optimal!

Yes, some people do need a low or very low carb count to get anything moving - the whole heap of genetics, gland health, previous dieting history, non-optimal gut microbiome that comes with life means their bodies need a more strict carbohydrate restriction to shift the fat- but not everyone does, so why cause "counting angst" to more people than required?

Ketosis is not some delicate flower - it's one of many processes that our body fluctuates between constantly -

and when we remove all the refined carbs, it resets back to managing itself properly again.

Unless there is a solid medical reason for being deeply ketogenic, moving back and forward between ketosis and brief periods of glucosis/glycosis in response to small amounts of fibre wrapped carbs in their natural state is natural to the human body - and by extension of the logic, helps us maintain a healthy metabolism so it deals well with whatever comes its way. Mark Sisson calls this "being on the bubble" and I agree with his view point entirely.

I also found this blog post by Amy Berger that says everything on this topic that I wished I'd written because I 100% agree with it as well.
http://www.tuitnutrition.com/2016/12/ketogenic-diet-rant.html

Think about it; you don't see the remaining hunter gatherer tribes still not following a westernised diet "watching what they eat and measuring their ketones" - they just eat food from the bounty of nature and thrive on it.

If you want to be keto or strict keto, you feel happy there and it suits your life, then go for it. But I personally don't think that you are doing yourself any favours over the long haul.

And yes, my opinion is simply that, an opinion based on anecdotal reading of posts made my original Yahoo lists and then my Facebook group as well as the logic drawn from all the science I've read - it "counts for nothing" scientifically, correlation is not causation etc etc.

I base my opinion on my observations; I've seen over and over and over that if people stay at 20g they hit issues later on down the line.

Whatever you chose, it's your educated empowered choice having listened to your body and woken up your mind. And that's the way life is at its happiest.

Part four

Rule Britannia! Translations of "all the things" that might trip you up on the way

The United States and Great Britain are two countries separated by a common language.

- George Bernard Shaw

The main reason that I created the Low Carb in the UK website and mailing lists back in 2000 is because a great deal of the information about a low carb way of eating comes from the US, where they have a very different set of laws and general context for buying and consuming food than we do in the UK.

In the last 60 years, US marketers have sold the messages that "bigger is better", "fat is poison" and "sugar is good" to the America public:

❖ The average portion size is the US is now astronomical, at around ~50% larger than it was 40 years ago.[100]
❖ The American public have been trained to expect most food to be sweet, both sweet and savoury dishes! The level of sweetness they expect is also much sweeter than we would expect or want.
  o This sweetness manipulation is called "The Bliss Point" and US manufacturers manipulate their goods ruthlessly to hit this point, to make consumers buy more.
❖ And they have a prevalence of the slightly sweeter "High Fructose Corn syrup" rather than the more expensive sucrose as the sweetener of manufacturing choice.

---

[100]http://www.yourweightmatters.org/portion-sizes-changed-time/and
https://www.ncbi.nlm.nih.gov/pmc/articles/PMC1447051/

To add insult to injury, great swaths of the US have no access to fresh produce, so they have no other option but to keep eating junk processed foods!

For us, where for most of us (but not all[101]) it's tricky to not find fresh fruit and vegetables within a short walk - the UK ideal is within 500m[102]- and with most major supermarkets now offering delivery at reasonable cost to most places in the UK, (although supermarkets do cause their own issues in pushing out small independent greengrocers and butchers!) it's unthinkable to not have access to fresh produce.

Yet according to the U.S. Department of Agriculture (USDA), twenty-nine million Americans live in urban and rural "food deserts."

They define this as areas of low income where
- ❖ Rural dwellers that have to travel at least 10 miles to get to their nearest supermarket.
- ❖ City dwellers that have to travel at least a mile to get to their nearest supermarket.

In America, where the car is king, a 15-minute, one-mile drive doesn't seem unreasonable. But in densely populated cities such as Washington D.C. where owning a car simply isn't practical, that can mean having to take

---

[101]http://www.researchcatalogue.esrc.ac.uk/grants/L135251002/read

[102]http://www.independent.co.uk/news/uk/home-news/food-deserts-depriving-towns-of-fresh-fruit-and-vegetables-764804.html

hour-long bus rides in each direction to get to a supermarket, with full shopping bags in tow on the way back.[103]

So, this part is all about our differences and how to not get tripped up or bent out of shape over trying to find something we don't have or have a totally different name for in the UK

---

[103]http://www.gracelinks.org/blog/5755/america-s-healthy-food-access-problem-is-not-sustainable

The "Grass-fed" thing

The US have a massive issue around the quality of their livestock (not that they think of it like this!) - They mostly ranch their cows in huge "feedlots" situated in the dryer states rather than allow their cows to graze where the grass is as we do in the UK and Europe.[104]

They also are the home to the "mega farm" - horrendous intense farming practices that cram too many animals into a small amount of space that are dreadful in terms of animal welfare but enables "Big Food" to make food more cheaply.

Consequently, they grow huge amounts of wheat, dent corn and soy to feed the cows, pigs and poultry, to ensure consistency and the ability to feed constantly and get the animal to market as quickly as possible. This is one of the strong arguments in the US for vegetarianism – why grow wheat and other crops for cows and pigs, when we could grow it for humans?

However, this grain-based diet causes an unnatural balance of Omega 6 to Omega 3 fats in the cow's body fat, which makes them less healthy for humans to consume. So, there is a massive push for "grass-fed beef" in US low carb and paleo food books and articles, that naturally overflows to us in the UK, reading them. They also don't rear sheep in the quantities that Europe does – the US is beef and bacon obsessed!

---

[104] http://www.beefusa.org/beefindustrystatistics.aspx

However, if you walk into a UK butcher and ask for grass-fed beef or lamb, they are going to give you a very funny look indeed! This is because in the UK, we don't really have an issue with "grass-fed vs grain fed" - British and Irish cows mostly live in green fields and eat mostly hay in winter. British and Irish sheep and goats live on hillsides, and again feed on grass and vegetation in summer, hay in the winter.[105]

Yes, there may well be fed some "pellet" cereal based foods thrown in for "finishing", but it's not the animal's exclusive diet. We get more than enough rain and have plenty of pasturable land (land that cannot be ploughed for crops, but easily grows grass for ruminant animals) to provide fresh grass as feed for both meat animals and the ones that produce dairy.

Most of Northern Europe is also the same. Plenty of green fields and hill sides to raise cattle and sheep on. France and Italy in particular are obsessive about the quality of life their animals live.

Pigs are a bit different, as pigs eat food given by the farmers. Pigs are omnivores, with a very similar digestive tract to our own. They naturally consume both plants and animals and in the wild they are foragers, primarily eating leaves, roots, fruits, and flowers, in addition to some insects, small animals and fish.

---

[105]https://www.food.gov.uk/business-industry/farmingfood/animalfeed/what-farm-animals-eat

Until very recently, man's relationship to the pig was intimate; most people kept a pig (and some chickens) and fed it their kitchen scraps AKA pig swill. However, due to both changing population, city density and lack of gardens etc, we stopped doing this.

Until the early 2000's, in all schools there was a "pig bin" (I remember the one in my school) where we very effectively recycled our food waste out to farmers via our local councils to feed pigs.

However, health concerns around Foot and Mouth in 2001 (for us not the animals) led to the banning of feeding food waste to pigs.[106]. Pigs reared for the mass market are now fed a mostly cereal "pellet" diet of corn and soy with a whole bunch of vitamins and minerals added, which is a whole 'nother issue about food sustainability and rain forest devastation in itself![107]

Mass product poultry reared for food, or battery producing eggs also receive a cereal based diet, whereas free range chickens, and the eggs their product, receive this feed but can also forage their environment for greens, insects, worms and other things birds more naturally eat. As a consequence, a free range bird cost us a heck of a lot more! And this is a good thing - *Ask not why real food is so expensive, ask why junk food is so cheap*"

---

[106]https://www.theguardian.com/environment/2013/jul/14/food-waste-fed-to-pigs

[107] http://www.thepigidea.org

With the rise of "cheap food pressures" however, this previous model is changing. UK farmers are under pressure from supermarkets to produce cheap food and so are importing the principles of US intense farming for Pigs, Poultry and Cattle[108]

Poultry in particular are now almost exclusively being reared in the UK in over-crowded and soulless conditions. In fact, the industry's move to using the word "farmed" rather than "reared" for their animals to me speaks volumes about the lack of respect that these animals receive.

This is one reason why my philosophy is *"buy the best food you can afford in all areas"* – if it costs you more as a consumer, the vegetables generally have more vibrancy and animals will have had a better quality of life. Giving respect to the animals you eat means that they taste better and are better for the body.

And yes, I sound a touch like an advert for veganism right now, which is something that I won't ever be. Whilst I respect people that make that choice, I personally don't think either going vegan or increasing our reliance on intense farming are global answers.

As with everything, the answer is a subtle shade of something in between, with a whole host of human

---

[108]https://www.theguardian.com/environment/2017/jul/17/uk-has-nearly-800-livestock-mega-farms-investigation-reveals

responsibility we have around opening our eyes and minds for the sake of all life on planet earth.

Whilst I don't 100% agree with his views on food, I personally like US journalist Michael Pollan's spin on eating[109] - *'Eat food, not too much, mostly plants"* – he's a rabid advocate of eating real food that people cook themselves, using fresh produce as well as growing your own food as you can and being connected into knowing about the food chain and ensuring it produced top quality in the food it produces.

I know for me, the amount of vegetables on my plate usually outnumbers the amount of animal protein, even before I saw his documentary.[110]

I buy from my local butcher, farmer's market and greengrocer as much as I can. I know that I'm also lucky that I have the money and these resources available to me, and I'm deeply thankful for this.

Whilst intense farming is not as big of an issue in the UK as it is in the US yet, doing your bit by spending money on good quality food is good for everyone. Putting good food into your body leads to an even better version of optimal you and putting money directly into a farmer's pocket leads to better farming practices as well.

---

[109] https://en.wikipedia.org/wiki/In_Defense_of_Food

[110] https://www.facebook.com/Nikola.Anne.Howard/posts/1601478173274682

UK labelling laws and "net" carbs

The difference in labelling law between the US and the UK and the concept of "Effective" or "Net" Carbs is the main reason why I started the LCUK mailing list and website back in the year 2000.

As I said, when I first began eating a low carbohydrate diet in 1999, Tim gave me the 1992 UK Vermillion published version of "Dr Atkins' New Diet Revolution" (DANDR), - written by an American, for the American market, with the explanation on how you count carbs given in chapter 5.

For the UK version, the publisher did not edit this chapter to reflect our labelling laws, the description of how to measure carbohydrate intake reflects the US labelling system.

It was Atkins Nutritionals Inc that the created the concept of "Net carbohydrate" - it is the "total carbohydrate count net of fiber" (note the US spelling of 'fiber' vs 'fibre' in the UK).

I got very confused back in my early days of eating this way, especially when I was doing the calculations as Dr Atkins' says and ending up with foods that had negative carbs in them! That's when I started doing research about the US and UK differences which ultimately led on to where I am now and this book being in the world.

When I read the 2015 UK Robinson published "Real Meal Revolution", I was infuriated that it quotes the US system. As Professor Noakes is South African, where their food labelling laws don't require nutrient breakdown at all, this leads me to assume that the US market version was simply republished for the UK as is. Which is simply lazy!

As you can well imagine, I swore and yelled at my eReader when I found this flaw in such a new book! Why would I be swearing? Well, I'm sure that you can guess the reason, in the UK (and the EU, where UK standards originate) our labelling standards and laws are completely different to those applied in the US.

In the UK,
1) The energy in the food in both Kilojoules and Kilocalories must be displayed.
2) The label must express the nutrition information (energy value and amounts of nutrients) per 100g, per 100ml or per portion of the food.
3) The exact amount in grams (g) of
    fat,
      of which saturates,
    carbohydrate,
      of which sugars,
    protein
    salt
must be displayed.

The manufacturer can also choose to add in, on a voluntary basis, the amounts of one or more of the following: monounsaturated fats, polyunsaturated fats, polyols, starch, fibre and some vitamins or minerals counted as significant if they are also present in significant amounts as defined by the regulation.

No other nutrient or substance may be declared in the nutrition declaration, for instance, there must be no declaration of trans fat or cholesterol content, and there is a specific layout of all the nutrients required, as you will have seen on the bread label I added earlier in Shift 7 [111]

The EU defines carbohydrate as:

> *''carbohydrate' means any carbohydrate which is metabolised by humans, and includes polyols;"*

and fibre as

> *'carbohydrate polymers with three or more monomeric units which are neither digested nor absorbed in the human small intestine"*

As fibre is non-digestible by humans, legally they are counted separately and are not part of the total carbohydrate count.

Simply put, our labelling standard is already "net of fibre," so if you are looking at a food package that came from an EU country, there is no need for complex maths or any other mucking about.

Unless the food contains Polyols, a listed per 100g "total carbohydrate" count on a package of food is 100% of the

_____

[111]https://www.gov.uk/government/uploads/system/uploads/attachment_data/file/595961/Nutrition_Technical_Guidance.pdf

carbs we need to count. And because of the way we measure our food, we have no "hidden" carbs at all.

Polyols: I have already discussed how the body processes them in depth earlier – If the manufacturer chooses to list polyol content on a label, it is listed under Carbohydrate as they are digestible in the human gut.

So, why was the very confusing to us concept of "Net carbs" created in the first place?

It's due to the very whacky way that fiber (note US spelling) is measured by US FDA, and how US labelling regulations counts macronutrients for food labelling purposes. Unlike in the EU, US macronutrient counts are not measured or reported that accurately.

The FDA mandates that food is assessed accurately for the amount in grams of fat, protein, moisture and ash per serving (which can be any amount the manufacturer chooses), and *'Total carbohydrate is calculated by subtracting the weight of crude protein, total fat, moisture, and ash from the total weight of the sample of food."*

As you can see, the US obtain their carbohydrate count "by difference" not by measurement as we do.

It goes on to state that *"Dietary fiber must be listed as a subcomponent under total carbohydrate."* [112]

As we discussed above, the human gut cannot process fibre, which is why Atkins Nutritional Inc. created the concept of the "net carb" and so our American cousins subtract the fiber amount listed in the nutrition facts panel from the given carbohydrate count to give them their "net carb count".

As far as Polyols go, US labelling standard concerning them state *'The listing of sugar alcohol is required when a claim is made on the label or in labeling about sugar alcohol or sugars when sugar alcohols are present in the food."*

So, if US Low-carb food manufacturers don't make any claims about them they are allowed to simply ignore them! Or, they can say that polyols are non-digestible, tell you the count, but then exclude that from the total food values.

And for our US cousins, the bad news about how to count carbohydrate doesn't stop there.

To add insult to injury, US manufacturers are allowed to "hide" carbs away as any carbohydrate measurement where the serving is a total of 50 calories and under is legitimately allowed to be rounded down to the nearest gram by the manufacturer or producer.

---

[112] https://www.fda.gov/downloads/Food/GuidanceRegulation/UCM265446.pdf - Nutrition facts, page 25-32

i.e. one large egg has ~0.4g of Carbohydrate in it, but US food producers can list this as zero in any products made from whole eggs where the serving size would be 1 egg or less.

That 0.4g is an example of "hidden carbs" mentioned by our American cousins. And they will affect US Low-carb life if too many are unknowingly eaten!

As you can see, we have it miles better than our American cousins, however, unnecessary confusion has been caused due to extremely lazy editing by book publishers that don't convert food labelling law sections over to fit UK law.

This is a personal bug-bear of mine, as so many people ask about this – and my want to get this information out there is at the root of why I'm now serving the world in the way that I do.

Low carb substitutes for high carbohydrate products AKA fake junk food

Fake junk food is another American invention that the UK is increasingly importing, sometimes literally.

When the "second wave" of low carb hit the US in earnest with the release of "Dr Atkins' New Diet Revolution" in 1992 as well as "The Zone" (Barry Sears) and "Protein Power" (Drs Michael and Mary Dan Eades) in 1995, American food culture was moving away from home cooking and family eating meals together.

Instead the US food market at that time was moving towards "convenience for working mothers" and "sweet foods as snack" which mean that a whole bunch of enterprising food manufacturers made substitute foods to meet the needs of this market. Atkins himself founded Atkins Nutritionals, Inc. in 1989 to promote low-carbohydrate pre-packaged products to accompany his diet.

A whole host of low carb breads, cracker, bake mixes, shake mixes, sweets, chocolates, sweeteners, sugar free pancake and coffee syrups, meal replacement bars and ready-to-drink shakes sprang onto the US market.

Strangely, as far as I know, no one has ever produced a "low carb market" targeted ready meal. I'd guess in part because it could not be bulk manufactured cheaply.

These types of substitutes cater to the assumption that, as Sarah Mabbitt, owner of http://www.avidlite.co.uk says "*you may have problems sticking to it because you are missing your bars of chocolate, sweets, savoury snacks, bread, cakes, cookies etc and bored with the limited options in your local supermarket.*"

However, as I've discussed in shift 7 and key 7, using these types of product is non-optimal for the body and also serves to reinforce our old habit patterns, making it far easier to fall back into simply eating the real thing, which usually tastes a heck of a lot better anyway.

Anecdotally, people report that if they eat these types of product, it slows or stalls their progress, increases feeling of lethargy, brain fog and bloating. To some, their body gives them the same feedback loop as if the food had been the real carbohydrate laden version. And of course, we've already talked about the gut biome destroying and laxative effects of over-consumption of Polyols.

I used these products heavily the first time around, so I never got myself "out of the bread and snack habit" whereas when I restarted in 2010, with the education of both the first time and all the research I'd done, I now make the choice not to eat these products unless I have no other choice.

Hey, if I get stuck somewhere, and the only option is between an Atkins' ready shake (Chocolate is the only one I feel to be at all palatable) or a low-fat sandwich and a bag of crisps, I'll take the hit and have the shake as the more optimal of the choices available.

As with all food and using the freedom of the ONS scale, it's your choice to eat these or not.

US vs UK names for food

As the Irish writer George Bernard Shaw allegedly said: 'England and America are two countries divided by a common language'[113] and with many of the low carb recipes on the Internet coming from America, some translation is required!

I'm not going to have found them all, but here are the most common ingredients that need translating:

US name	UK name
Almond flour/meal	Ground almonds
Arugula	Rocket
Bacon	Streaky Bacon
Beet	Beetroot
Bell Pepper	Green, Red or Yellow peppers
Biscuits	A scone like product, slightly lighter in texture and made with almost no sugar
Broiler	Grill
Canadian Bacon	Back Bacon
Celery root	Celeriac
Cider	Apple juice
Cilantro	Coriander
Coconut butter	Creamed Coconut (the stuff we get in blocks)
Cookies	Biscuits
Corn starch	Cornflour

---

[113] It's also been attributed to Oscar Wilde and Winston Churchill

Crock Pot	Slow Cooker
Cutlet	Chop
Cupcake	Fairy Cake
Eggplant	Aubergine
English Muffin	Muffin
Frosting	Icing
Garbanzo beans	Chickpeas
Grill	Barbeque
Ground meat	Mince
Gyro	Kebab
Half and Half	No UK equivalent – this is a 10% dairy fat liquid, you can make it by mixing 50:50 Full fat milk to single cream
Hard Cider	Cider
Heavy Cream	Double Cream
Heavy Whipping cream	Whipping cream
Hot Sauce	Chilli sauce
Jell-O	Jelly
Light Cream	Single Cream
Light Whipping cream	No UK equivalent – use Single
Molasses	Treacle
Muffins	American Muffin - Overly large cupcakes, usually made with oil and either berries, nuts or chocolate chips
Oatmeal	Porridge
Pot	Saucepan
Powdered Sugar	Icing Sugar

Pudding	A type of gloopy dessert, a bit like Angel delight.
Rutabaga	Swede (Yellow Turnip or 'Neep if you are a Scot)
Scallion	Spring Onion
Shredded Coconut	Desiccated Coconut
Shrimp	Prawn
Skillet	Frying Pan
Swiss Chard	Chard or Rainbow Chard
Virginia Ham	Gammon
White Raisins (Or Golden Raisins)	Sultanas
Zucchini	Courgette

A word on the differences in cuts of meat

Meat cuts in the UK and the US (and also most of the rest of the world!) are not only differently named, they come from different bits of the Animal! So, it's difficult, but not impossible to translate UK cuts to US recipes

So, I'm going to link over to Wikipedia, cos it gives you much more information that I could ever convey here without plagiarising someone else's information!

Beef:
https://en.wikipedia.org/wiki/Cut_of_beef

Pork:
https://en.wikipedia.org/wiki/Cut_of_pork

Lamb and Mutton:
https://en.wikipedia.org/wiki/Lamb_and_mutton#Cuts

US vs UK food measuring

And as much as our language separates us, the way that US and UK recipes are constructed is also different.

Rather than using weight to measure ingredients, as most of the rest of the world does, Americans measure their ingredient quantities by volume when cooking. either by the teaspoon, tablespoon or "cup" measurement.

Officially a US cup is 240ml and a metric cup, widely available here and also Australia and South Africa is 250ml. However, as the use of the cup as a measurement in any recipe is proportional, using a metric cup gives no difference at all to the result.

As an interesting side note, if you ever cook from an Australian recipe, their tablespoons are 20ml, not 15ml like the rest of the world!

The US also has its own system of weights and measures - the "US customary measurement system" which is based on British Imperial measurement standard before 1824.[114]

The only noteworthy thing for cooking is that a US pint is only 16 Fl oz, not 20 like the UK pint.

---

[114]https://en.wikipedia.org/wiki/Comparison_of_the_imperial_and_US_customary_measurement_systems

A US Fl. Oz is also ever so slightly larger than the Imperial Fl oz, but the difference is so small as to not really be noticeable.

I found that buying myself a set of measuring spoons and cups was the easiest solution for the American recipes, and I now actually much prefer cooking in cups and spoons, unless I'm needing the accuracy for the cooking chemistry. I find that it's generally easier than weighing, even if it does create more washing up.

American recipes for desserts and confections – reduce the sweetener!

Talking of cooking, if you are following a US dessert or sweet recipe, remember that most of our American cousins are still looking for the same level of sweetness to which they are accustomed. As I mentioned above, American food manufacturers have a great deal riding on an elevated "bliss point" for the public!

Consequently, for most US recipes, you can usually cut the amount of sweetener required by at least a third, if not by half. I'd always advise when trying a new recipe to make it "as is" on the first go, and then tweak it to how you want it going forward.

However, for US sweet recipes, I always cut down on the sweetener on the first go. Also remember that as your low carb journey carries on, your own "bliss point" level will drop and you will want food to be less sweet in any case.

You made it!

Welcome to the rest of your life!

Excellence is an art won by training and habituation. We do not act rightly because we have virtue or excellence, but we rather have those because we have acted rightly. We are what we repeatedly do. Excellence, then, is not an act but a habit.

-    Aristotle

Well done, you've now changed your way of eating and are also well on the way to changing the way you think as well!

I trust that I've now armed you with a new outlook on food, your body, your mind and your life.

Ongoing support is vital to success, so why not join my Low Carb in the UK Facebook group:

http://tiny.cc/LCUKFBG

Or if you feel that you would like some more individual advice, I'm on coach.me for digital mentoring & coaching.

https://www.coach.me/NikolaHoward?ref=ZM0PW

Use the coupon NIKOLAHOWARDWEEK for a free week of digital coaching

Free gifts: Printables supplement and subliminal audio bonus

I understand that journaling to an empty page can be daunting, especially if you have not done it before, so any exercises that I've suggested you complete I've given sample structure for in the supplement.

Also, this is where you will find around 55 recipes, formatted so that they don't break across pages, so that they can be easily printed and used in the kitchen!

I've also created a 20 minutes subliminal audio for you. Subliminal audio is used to transform old, unwanted habits or thinking patterns that are stubbornly stuck in the subconscious.

Play the audio in the background at low volume as much as you feel comfortable, although it is suggested that subliminal audios should be used for around one hour per day for a minimum of 30 days for best effect.

As the audio is 20 minutes long, this means that playing it in the background of whatever you are doing 3 times a day will do the job.

Although you can play it more as you wish, if you play it all the time, this might result in overload to your subconscious. Overload will often result in a person's mind refusing to accept the positive reinforcement, which is naturally counterproductive to the success I want you to have!

Go to the webpage below (either use your phone to scan the QR code or type the address into your web browser) and use the password "**YesToSuccess!**" to access the sign-up form that will send you your gifts via email.

http://tiny.cc/HTDLCUKS-Gifts

The page will collect your details so that I know where to send your gifts and will also ask you if you wouldn't mind me sending you updates, hints tips and other stuff that I don't share anywhere else.

Acknowledgements

This book has been kicking around in my head since 2005 or so - I even drafted an outline for it in 2010, which then promptly got packed in a box and put in storage, as I was doing a complete house renovation! So, I'm happy that it is finally escaping my brain and is out into the world helping people.

Firstly, my thanks to Tim Brutton, the chap that introduced me to "Dr Atkins' New Diet Revolution" in Spring 1999. Without you having read the book yourself and then passing it onto me because you thought it might help, I would probably not be living a low carb life and never be writing this book!

An honourable mention goes out to the members of the original LCUK Yahoo! mailing list, in particular; Joanne, Jeanette, Katy, Kevin and Lilian. Without them and the other members to bounce my fears, worries and triumphs off, I would never have made the website that turned into http://www.lowcarbinthe.uk in August 2000.

I must also acknowledge the work of Barry Groves PhD and its effects on me and my thinking. Now sadly deceased, Barry was a man that I feel deeply privileged to have known personally, and his work and deep love of all the science influenced me heavily. He gave tirelessly of his time and knowledge to the world through his own books, websites and speaking tours.

He spent many hours on the LCUK and CLCUK Yahoo! mailing lists helping both myself and other members understand the science behind the Low Carbohydrate way of eating and shining a light for the UK when there was no one else doing so.

A big shout out to Manette and Emma, who allowed me to interview them for their experiences with a low carb life and their stories helped to build the narrative bits of this book, even if I didn't use them in the end.

My thanks also to all members of the LCUK Facebook group, for their inspiration, recipes and general cheerleading as I slogged my way through the difficult to write sections.

My eternal gratitude goes out to the current moderator team; Katy, Lisa and Lilian, as well as ex-moderators Jessica and Joanne. They've allowed me to write distraction free when I've needed to and kept me on track when I've posted too much in the group when I should have been writing this instead!

Finally, to everyone that pre-ordered this book. It wouldn't be in the world without you. Self-publishing is awesome, but research, graphics and ISBN numbers aren't cheap. I'm humbled that 117 people had faith in me to write this book and bring it into the world.

THANK YOU!

Printed in Great Britain
by Amazon

45473261R00203